Top Ten Tips for Tip Top Shape

Top Ten Tips for Tip Top Shape

Super Health Programs

For All Professional Fields

- Service - Healthcare - Education - Legal - Manufacturing - Retail -

Any Many More!

Matthew DeLeo and Douglas Haddad

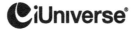

Top Ten Tips for Tip Top Shape
Super Health Programs For All Professional Fields

iUniverse books may be ordered through booksellers or by contacting:

iUniverse
1663 Liberty Drive
Bloomington, IN 47403
www.iuniverse.com
1-800-Authors (1-800-288-4677)

Because of the dynamic nature of the Internet, any web addresses or links contained in this book may have changed since publication and may no longer be valid. The views expressed in this work are solely those of the author and do not necessarily reflect the views of the publisher, and the publisher hereby disclaims any responsibility for them.

Any people depicted in stock imagery provided by Thinkstock are models, and such images are being used for illustrative purposes only. Certain stock imagery © Thinkstock.

Top Ten Tips for Tip Top Shape is intended to provide helpful and informative material for healthy adults, ages 18 and over. This book does not provide medical advice. Please consult a medical or health professional before you engage in any new exercise, nutrition, supplementation or wellness program.

The authors specifically disclaim all responsibility for any liability or losses, personal or otherwise, that is included as a consequence, directly or indirectly, of the use and application of any of the information that is provided in this book.

ISBN: 978-0-5953-4932-6 (sc)
ISBN: 978-0-5957-9646-5 (e)

Print information available on the last page.

iUniverse rev. date: 03/30/2017

CONTENTS

ACKNOWLEDGMENTS

Working on this project, we encountered many obstacles in our path as anyone would and there are special people that we would like to thank among the many for their endearing support in the development and production of our debut book. We want to thank these individuals for helping us achieve our goals:

-Jack & Carol DeLeo and Mike & Donna Haddad for supporting us ALWAYS

-Jennie DeLeo, Mike DeLeo, Dawn D'Angelo, Joe & Clare Petrucelli and Joe J. Petrucelli as continued bodies of support and inspiration throughout our lives

-our teachers in school that demonstrated great patience and believed in us growing up

-Sarah, Laurie, Julie, Jill, Jakki, Bill and the 300+ clients who utilized and benefited from the customized fitness plans for success

-John Mitchell (BBPics Photography, www.bbpics.com), our photographer for the book, who is a great friend of ours and a tremendous source of encouragement for all of our projects

-Norman Savanella for dedicating his time in graphically constructing much of the design of our book

-Manhattan Fitness for granting us permission to conduct the exercise photo session

-Mark Modine for taking time out of his busy schedule to demonstrate different exercises exhibited in the book

-the Westport wiseguys (the best of the best): Berkowitz, Pauly B., Howard, the M & M boys (Marvin and Murray Lender)

-a special young lady who "let Doug fly" years ago to achieve his destiny and one that will fly along beside him in the future. You are with me my dear "bug girl"!

CHAPTER 1

ROCK AND ROLL INTRO

In what direction is our society headed? We are living in a fast-paced highly competitive society where we as Americans often choose to neglect our bodies. Yet, all of us have an innate desire to want to look and feel our best, but for the most part we fail. This is just plain ridiculous!

Sadly enough, there is a growing trend in our society where more individuals are becoming obese by the day. In fact, more than 65 % of Americans are considered overweight. As you can clearly see, this is a daily problem. There seems to be a quest to shed those unwanted pounds with as little effort as possible in the shortest stint of time. The goal is to acquire a desired state of health, but at what cost? Does this sound oxymoronic (generating an increased health state by doing long term damage to your body)? The two just do not coincide.

Over 50 million Americans will go on some sort of diet program and only a mere 5-10% succeed and achieve their goals for a given period of time contributing to the staggering $40 billion in revenue amassed by the weight loss industry annually. Many of these diets and weight loss products make claims such as "rapid weight loss", "no diet or exercise required", "eat whatever you want and lose the weight". These are hot buttons that these advertisers use to get us to spend $800 (avg.) for their products and services. If it sounds too good to be true, it probably is.

We need to understand that we have control over our physical and mental well beings. Often times we are plagued by the daily pressures that tend to consume us. Moreover, we feel that we do not have enough time in a day to dedicate towards improving physical as well as mental strength. There are deceptive advertisements that do not address a person's specific goals and fitness aspirations. Our book, *Top Ten Tips for Tip Top Shape* offers a wide range of customized plans that can be followed daily at work and at home. There isn't any "finding time to workout". It can be achieved with some basic understanding of your lifestyle.

Whatever your profession may be, there is a specific plan that will work for you. What may work for a computer programmer may not work the same for a plumber. We account for varying activity levels, stress levels, hours worked, & other time constraints. No matter what occupation you work at, we show you tips that will help you achieve your fitness & wellness goals.

How can you be certain that the designed plan works specifically for YOU? As we understand each person's own unique differences within the same profession, we also realize that it comes down to the belief and motivation of the individual, when given the proper set of directions and tools to work with, to achieve his/her goals. We have worked on a one-to-one basis with individuals from all of these professions and we have seen outstanding results achieved time and time again. Your profession plays a very important role in your overall wellness. We have outlined 20 specific customized programs to suit your needs. These plans are designed with a long-term intention for a healthy lifestyle. You may have some concerns and come across some obstacles that stand in your way in your desire to achieve a healthier lifestyle. Here are the top ten concerns that our clients have expressed to us.

10. *I come home from work and never feel like I have enough energy to go to the gym. My work takes all of my energy and time.*

9. *I go all day without eating because I simply don't have time. I am so consumed with my work.*

8. *I never get enough sleep at night.*

7. *I work 10-hour days and never have time to work out with all of the other things I have to do after work.*

6. *On the weekends, all I want to do is watch TV, drink beer, and relax.*

5. *I end up eating late at night everyday because of my hectic schedule.*

4. *I am bored with my job and hence I am never motivated to go to the gym.*

3. *I travel all of the time and eat out at restaurants frequently.*

2. *The cafeteria foods at work are not nutritious.*

1. *I have to sit at my desk all day and my hips keep getting bigger.*

Do these concerns sound familiar? We address these concerns and obstacles in your own customized program and give you the ammunition you will need to attack these issues. Ask yourself, "Is my goal to improve my physical and mental well beings using a plan that does work in a time efficient manner?" If your goals range from improving your physique to being in tip top shape or to feeling your best and looking your best in the workplace, then this is it. These chapters ahead will provide you with a plan of attack that is ageless! This is the only book that you will need 1, 5, 10, 20, 30 years from now. We focus on you and your lifestyle and critique it for methods on how to get one step at a time closer to SUPER HEALTH.

The time for excuses is over! There are no more excuses to be had. Whether you are young of age or like most of working America (or retired) where time unfortunately waits for no one, you will be able to realistically implement a personalized plan for sustained health. Here are our top ten reasons for creating our book and why these innovative customized SUPER HEALTH programs will work for you.

10. *Creativity Levels*

Some professions such as architects, graphic designers, and various scientists work with the left side of their brain analyzing different problems, and other people are more right-sided thinkers where spatial aptitude ability is very high (ex. sculptors, artists, writers, etc.). A set, rigid nutrition formula may not work for both sets of professions so we have different, specialized creative workouts right for each professional field.

9. *On and Off Levels*

Politicians, public speakers, salesmen, teachers, television personalities, etc. have to be "on" the majority of the day at work to be successful. Other professions in manufacturing, production, retail, etc. are sometimes forced to turn it "off". We show you how you can always be "on" or at least make the day more active in the face of monotony.

8. *Travel Time & Income Levels*

If you are racking up those frequent flier miles or simply "on the road again", then you will learn how you can eat right and work out away from home to maximize your wellness.

7. *Activity Levels: High? Low? Medium?*

We cover all spectra, from the sedentary worker's daily activity level to the manual laborer's who may be getting his/her fair share of exercise at work.

6. *Standing or Sitting*

This makes a difference in your daily caloric expenditure. Active movement in some form or fashion is a must to get you on a healthy track. There are a great deal of professions that lack that minimal daily movement so we address the "moving more" philosophy head on.

5. *Stress & Anxiety Levels*

These two factors translate into many unfortunate health risks. Each profession deals with certain stress-related incidents (some more pressing than others). Stress can accumulate and impact one's lifestyle and we advise tips for relieving the stress levels and moving forward in a more health-conscious manner.

4. *Different Personalities*

Intense personalities (type A) need intense workouts that have set schedules. Relaxed, more laid back types (type B) will require something varied & not so rigid in schedule. We provide just the right ingredients for these types.

3. *Different Motivations & Goals*

We all work off of different hot buttons so what motivates a chef to perform may greatly contrast that for an entrepreneur. Even people of the same age & gender can vary significantly. A 40-year old female secretary's goals & lifestyle most likely differ from that of a 40-year old female waitress' goals. We set up strategies where you can excel in your profession as well as reach peak fitness levels.

2. *Too much time spent at work*

Your profession may require 12-hour days versus the standard 8-hour shift. Just finding the time to work out would be an accomplishment. We show you how you can incorporate a workout into your hectic schedule. Three hours out of a typical 112 weekly awake hours is all it takes to retrieve higher energy levels and physical wellness.

1. *Different shifts*

As you know, not all professions have the typical 9-5 P.M. shift. Many policemen, firemen, EMTs, and physicians are on the clock 24 hours a day, 7 days a week. We show you the best times to work out to maximize your physical and mental benefits based on when you are awake and available.

All 10 of these reasons play a major factor in your physical and mental wellness. We took into consideration these reasons when we designed your customized program for you in your professional field. This book captures the profiles of 20 different professions and how in great detail, we explain the dos and don'ts of each profession. This is what makes our book unique, timely and innovative. Its intent is to look at over 95% of different occupations focusing on over 120 million people and having each person follow his/her own personalized workout routine, proper food intake level, lifestyle tips, etc. Lifestyle-altering diets and excessive exercising are not the answer. We will show you how to make consistent daily decisions that will benefit you long term and inevitably result in what many individuals claim to be "bodily miracles".

We feel confident that the information provided will be beneficial for all. One size doesn't fit all so we incorporate specialized workouts and diets based on the different factors of your profession. We have worked on a one-to-one basis with people of all ages, all body types, and levels of motivation, and all types of professions, helping them reach their physical goals as well as enhancing their mental well being. The goal of this book is not just to develop a better physique, but furthermore to gain a personal awareness that if you can achieve this viable task of "SUPER HEALTH" with a plan, then you can achieve anything in this life with a plan.

We enjoy providing people with the power of knowledge to change their lives for the better. No matter what job or career you are currently working in, we have the "SUPER HEALTH" program for you. For instance, if you are a male accountant, then the WHITE-COLLAR professional field is where you will look for your customized program. If you are a female and work in a bake shop, then the RETAIL AND GROCERY professional field is where your "SUPER HEALTH" program resides.

It is as easy as that. Look under our 20 professional fields that we list here and find out where your job fits in. And this folks is where your own customized 'SUPER HEALTH' program is. Follow the tips mentioned in your own program and you will be on your way to realize the type of physical and mental well being that you have always dreamed of. Go get em!

20 DIFFERENT PROFESSIONAL FIELDS

1. OVER 55 & RETIREES

2. COMPUTER RELATED
1. IT tech
2. Web programmers
3. Computer technology
4. Consultants

3. DELIVERY DRIVERS & POSTAL
1. Postal employees
2. Fedex, UPS
3. Local delivery drivers
4. Limo/taxi drivers
5. Bus drivers

4. EDUCATION
1. Teachers (k-12)
2. Administrators
3. Professors (college)
4. Counselors
5. Coaches

5. HEALTHCARE
1. Physicians
2. EMS, on call doctors
3. Nurses
4. Surgical Technicians
5. Private practice physicians, therapist
6. Specialized doctors(ex. dentists, gynecologists, obstetricians)

6. HIGH PROFILE
1. Politicians
2. Media personnel (TV, radio)
3. Actors, musicians & models
4. Public speakers

7. HIGH LEVEL RESPONSIBILITY
1. CEOs, presidents, upper level mngt.
2. Wall Street & brokerage firms
3. Business owners, GMs

8. HOTEL & RESTAURANT
1. Fast food employees
2. Hotel personnel
3. Chefs & cooks
4. House cleaners
5. Waiters, waitresses, bartenders

9. LAW ENFORCEMENT & FIREMEN
1. Policemen
2. Firemen
3. Detectives, secret service
4. Security guards, bodyguards

10. LEGAL
1. Lawyers & attorneys
2. Judges
3. Paralegals

11. MANUFACTURING & PRODUCTION
1. Manufacturing
2. Warehouse
3. Machine operators
4. Shipping & receiving
5. Linework

12. PINK COLLAR JOBS (women)
1. Secretaries, receptionists
2. Admin assistants & clerical
3. Corporate employees
4. Banking & finance
5. Bookkeepers

13. RETAIL & GROCERY
1. Cashiers & baggers
2. Stockers
3. Deli & bakery
4. Produce/meat/seafood
5. Customer service

14. RIGHT SIDE OF THE BRAIN JOBS
1. Architects
2. Computer-aided draftsmen
3. Journalists & writers
4. Engineers
5. Interior decorators & designers
6. Painters & sculptors

15. SALES & MARKETING
1. Entrepreneurs, self-employed
2. Salesmen
3. Marketing
4. Agents (ex. real estate, sports, private)
5. Advisors & directors

16. SERVICE JOBS
1. Cosmetologists & beauticians
2. Personal trainers & lifeguards
3. Massage therapists
4. Hairstylists
5. Private instructors (ex. voice coaches)

17. SKILLED MANUAL LABOR
1. Landscaping
2. Building & construction, carpentry
3. Electricians, HVAC, plumbers
4. Custodians
5. Automotive technicians

18. STAY AT HOME MOMS
1. Pre & post natal

19. TRAVEL
1. Cross country truck drivers
2. Pilots
3. International positions
4. Correspondents
5. Stewards/stewardesses

20. WHITE-COLLAR JOBS (men)
1. Corporate employees
2. Accountants
3. Banking & finances
4. Business
5. Analysts

CHAPTER 2

TOP TEN TOOLS FOR EACH PROFESSION

Every profession has its own set of tools for success. Your personalized "SUPER HEALTH" plan has its own set of tools that you can keep in your back pocket to help you achieve your wellness goals. Take these 10 tools to work with you every day:

10. *EMBRACE CHALLENGES*

The human body is made to accept challenges and respond to adversity. It adapts to stress mentally, physically, and emotionally. Continue to challenge your body mentally and physically. Start with small challenges and try to conquer them first. Success breeds success and as you surmount small hurdles, the bigger hurdle will be conquered before you know it. Overcoming obstacles equals triumph and re-setting the bar for you. You will accomplish what you never thought possible by embracing these challenges with confidence.

9. *GET MOVING*

We state this tool with a strong emphasis to the current American lifestyle. The key to achieving most fitness goals is to move more and eat less. Over 120 million people in America are overweight. This number is steadily increasing year-by-year. Whenever possible at work, running errands, or at home choose to move more for a healthier and better you.

8. *A COMPETITIVE MENTAL EDGE*

The saying goes that there is always someone working that much harder than you out there. Does that mean that you have to be number 1 at everything you do? No, but never settle for 2nd. Do the best that you can and set your own level of excellence. In sports, coaches & instructors drive home this concept of mental toughness. The greatest athletes and leaders today have one thing in common that drives them: a highly competitive drive to be the best. Take this mentality with you to work, the gym, home, everywhere.

7. *INSPIRATIONS*

What the mind perceives, it can do. Remember that all of the great heroes of our time had past failures and all of the "experts" in their crafts were once "beginners". Keep inspiring pictures, signs, and sayings at work to remind you of where you want to go in life. Remember the significant people that you have met that believed in you. They believed in you for a reason. There are momentous events in a person's life that inspire him or her to achieve. Sometimes a negative experience can be your biggest inspiration (someone telling you that you look like you put on a few pounds!). Turn these experiences into positives and use it as fuel to get your act in high gear. Life is too succinct to dwell on what could have been. Be an inspiration yourself and make it happen!

6. *BE MENTALLY TOUGH*

Any fear that you have is a learned fear and therefore can be erased. Fear can be the wall around your paradise. It can squash the human spirit if overplayed in one's mind on a consistent basis like a pre-recorded message. A wise man once told us, "If it were easy, EVERYONE would do it!" Believe in yourself and visualize attaining those physical and mental wellness levels like never before. You may not get the desired support that you want or deserve. You may not achieve your goals on schedule. Don't take the easy way out and quit, but instead resolve the situation, make adjustments necessary and go again. Have that "try-again" mentality. Your time **will** come and you will be an unbelievable inspiration for many of the non-believers.

5. *HAVE A POSITIVE ATTITUDE*

Look at the 24 oz. bottle of water that you are about to drink as half-FULL. Be proactive and take control of your body. Positive things happen to positive people. These people are shown to enjoy life to a much greater extent and experience a healthy state of mind and body. Tell yourself that you can do something and then figure out how you can get it done. The six-inch space that you possess between your cranium contains the formula for success. Go find it!

4. *STAY FOCUSED ON YOUR GOALS*

Identify what it is that you want. Formulate a plan to achieve these goals. There will be many detours along the path, which could interfere with obtaining your goals. Keep the fire burning strongly, stay patient and analyze your progress. If you don't see any progress, ask yourself the question, "WHY?" You may need to make adjustments along the road to your goals, but stay true to what you want. It is the accumulation of hard work and executing your plan that wins out in the long run. When you hit one of your goals, reward yourself for the achievement and get re-focused again for future successes.

3. *PASSION AND INTENSITY*

Do everything with passion and intensity and soon you will have the extra something that you can call upon to achieve your goals. Others will notice this flame burning brightly inside of you resonating loudly, and respect will follow. Have a great work ethic and devote your pride into what you do and your best will shine!

2. *SET GOALS*

A goal is nothing more than a dream with a deadline. You have to set goals in order to be a high achiever. It is like climbing the ladder of success one step at a time. Eighty percent of the goals that are written down on paper come true. Set weekly, monthly, yearly goals, both short-term and long-term. You want to know where you are going, where you want to end up and how you will get there. By setting goals, you can help manifest your destiny. Make these goals clear, specific, and attainable. You want to challenge yourself, but be realistic also. Dreaming is good, but be aware that lofty short-term goals can be a recipe for failure.

Weekly goals:
> Ex. Get 4 workouts in this week
> Ex. Cook and prepare my all-star foods
> Ex. Do 50 pushups a day
> Ex. Challenge myself in 2 new ways this week

Monthly goals:
> Ex. Lose 3 lbs. fat and put on 1 lb muscle
> Ex. Take my work to the next level
> Ex. Increase my bench press 10 lbs.
> Ex. Get consistent nightly rest of 8 hours

Yearly goals:
> Ex. Reduce body fat from 22% to 15%
> Ex. Develop 10 new challenges (5-physically, 5-mentally)
> Ex. Read 5 mind-stimulating books
> Ex. Improve in a particular sport
> Ex. Alter my eating patterns to include all-star foods as part of my diet 80% of the time

1. *BE CONSISTENT*

Develop good habits and realize that you are doing this for the greater good of yourself. It takes 21 straight days to create a habit. Focus carefully on making them good habits. Bad habits don't miraculously disappear by themselves. You must work to undo them and then substitute them with something more positive that is part of your goals. Try your best at everything you do. That's all that you can ask of yourself and that is all that is asked of you. Success is a marathon of sorts. Slow and steady wins the race rather than a haphazard sprint to the finish line.

CHAPTER 3

TOP TEN RESULTS FOR EACH PROFESSION

We get you the results that you are looking for. Here are our Top 10 results that you will see by following your own SUPER HEALTH programs for your profession.

10. *MENTALLY STRONGER*

Getting in shape and staying in shape may be one of the biggest accomplishments in your life and this will result in you being mentally tough. Achieving this challenging fitness goal is a symbol of your character. You have the power to achieve anything that you truly put your mind to.

9. *BETTER RESULTS AT WORK*

You will have gained an extra energy and vitality from your wellness. Your work will benefit greatly. Your positive attitude will be recognized and pay increases and upward mobility may appear that much easier.

8. *MAKE YOUR LOVED ONES HAPPIER*

First and foremost, you will feel proud of yourself and you can focus on others company with great pleasure. Your happiness will rub off on others around you. That special someone will greatly benefit from your resounding zest for life. Your intimacy will be much greater and your partner will be more attracted to this positive, upbeat, energetic attitude.

7. *IMPROVED LIFESTYLE*

This is the ultimate goal of this book! Obtaining a self-actualization of what you can do and hopefully what you WILL do. Think long-term of what you most desire and translate that into short steps that will get you there.

6. *INCREASED HAPPINESS*

You will develop a healthier and happier way about you through consistent training. Happiness is a byproduct of hard work rewarded with results. Being mentally and physically strong is a reagent for jubilance. In the end, there is truly no other formula for happiness than to do what you love and love what you do!

5. *MORE CONFIDENCE*

Belief in one self can carry you to great places. Make strides every day to do your best and soon enough success will follow. When the other results begin to unfold as they may, you will realize that you actually can do it! Your self-esteem and confidence will bring you to a new dimension of "reality" that is yours and yours alone.

4. *STRONGER BONES AND MUSCLES*

We can delay the aging process tremendously with proper exercise. Our muscles become 10% weaker each decade if we don't train them properly. Hence, this being one of the biggest reasons we have to engage in a resistance training/cardiovascular program.

3. *HELPS PREVENT MANY DISEASES*

Science may not be able to solve all of the health-related concerns about different conditions that people can acquire throughout their lifetime. The pharmaceutical industry generates billions upon billions of dollars a year in profit selling various types of drugs for different diseases. With today's knowledge about discovered toxicity in various prescription drugs, the best cure for disease is prevention and educating the public about this. Science may not be able to capture the complete benefits of exercise and fitness, either. "A pound of prevention is worth an ounce of cure."

2. *LOOK BETTER, FEEL BETTER, & SLEEP BETTER*

Everything correlates to a better you! Practice makes perfect and getting into healthy habits of working out regularly, eating all-star foods, and getting good, consistent sleep nightly will have a compounding beneficial effect. Your outlook on waking up and facing the world will be brighter and staying focused on working harder will be that much easier.

1. *ACHIEVING **SUPER HEALTH** AND OVERALL WELLNESS*

Need we say more?

CHAPTER 4

TOP TEN TIPS FOR EACH PROFESSION

We break down every profession using the following Top Ten Tips and a section called 'It's part of the job'. These tips make it easy, clear and concise to understand and implement into your daily routine.

IT'S PART OF THE JOB

1.   The stress level of the job
2.   The activity level of the job
     - We provide a rating scale (1-10), 1-least active/stressful to 10-most active/stressful.
     - These two factors play important roles in customizing programs and assigning different types of food to eat & avoid.
3.   Time constraints
     - We discuss strategies on when to eat and workout within your busy day. We work with your energy levels, mentality, and attitude during the optimal times of the day when you will most benefit.

10. *LIFESTYLE TIPS*

1.   We overview a synopsis of your daily lifestyle.
2.   We discuss how you can make minor changes in your lifestyle to obtain major health benefits.
3.   Tips applied into your lifestyle will enhance your productiveness at work all around.
4.   We summarize how you can obtain "SUPER HEALTH" by implementing our tips.

9. *ALL-STAR FOODS & LIQUID FUEL*

1.   We offer a variety of different foods to be eaten (based on your profession)
     a.   Foods at home
     b.   Foods at work

      c.   Foods on the road (ex. "Fit Fast Foods")

      d.   Liquid fuel

2.   You must eat well 80% of the time (80/20 rule) to achieve any wellness and fitness goals.

3.   Sources of foods come from complex carbohydrates, lean sources of protein, and healthy fats.

4.   Water is the medium in which most cellular activities take place, including the transport and oxidation of lipids (fat), muscle-building process, and energy formation.

8. *FOODS TO AVOID*

1.   We discuss foods that should be eaten rather infrequently, those in lesser portions, and foods that should be completely avoided.

2.   Many of the foods having a higher glycemic index and a high level of saturated fat/trans fat are discussed as foods to avoid.

7. *MEALS: HOW MANY & WHEN*

1.   When you eat during the day makes a big difference toward your goals.

      a.   Breakfast is the most important meal of the day.

      b.   Small balanced meals should be eaten throughout the day at regular time intervals.

2.   We discuss how you can bring your all-star food choices with you to work and set up a schedule for eating (even during those hectic days).

3.   When eating at the correct times, you maximize the thermal effect of the food.

6. *SUPPLEMENTATION & SLEEP*

1.   The supplement industry is booming with tons of new supplements on the market each day. The FDA does not regulate this industry.

2.   We recommend the supplements that will help an individual in his/her profession reach his/her wellness goals.

3.   We rate these supplements in another chapter discussing the benefits claimed for each product, a top tip, and a rating of its benefit exclusively for you.

4.   We discuss which supplements should be part of your daily intake (A-List-primary, B-List-secondary)

5.   The all-important 8-hours of sleep is essential for children and is required for adults of all ages. This is often times overlooked as a key factor in achieving a healthy state of being.

5. *RESISTANCE TRAINING*

1.   This is the key to altering your physique and increasing your metabolism.

2.   We design a customized weight-training program for each profession. The workout is goal-specific and designed to:

      a.   enhance productivity & energy levels at work
      b.   reduce your stress & anxiety levels
      c.   increase your muscle strength & endurance

3.   Each program is designed with a certain intensity in mind. We provide a % failure one should try to reach in the workout to achieve a peak physique. Overloading the muscle is important to recruit new muscle fibers into action.

NOTE: We realize that individual differences must be accounted for so check with a physician before attempting these exercises. The number of sets/repetitions for an exercise can be adjusted based on personal fitness levels.

4.   We discuss the advantages of resistance training:
      a.   builds muscle, strengthens bones, ligaments, & your nervous system
      b.   promotes psychological well being
      c.   helps control your body weight
      d.   energy expenditure is elevated for 2-15 hours after your workout
      e.   energy demands are increased by using more calories during this timeframe
      f.   helps reduce your body fat levels

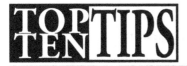

BODY FAT PERCENTAGE SCALE

The following table below provides a rating system for evaluating one's current body fat and fitness levels.

MALES

AGE	RISKY	EXCELLENT	GOOD	FAIR	POOR	VERY POOR
19-24	<6%	10.7%	14.9%	19.0%	23.3%	>23.3%
25-29		12.8%	16.5%	20.3%	24.4%	
30-34		14.5%	18.0%	21.5%	25.2%	
35-39		16.2%	19.4%	22.6%	26.2%	
40-44		17.5%	20.5%	23.6%	26.9%	
45-49		18.6%	21.8%	24.5%	27.6%	
50-54		19.8%	22.7%	25.6%	28.7%	
55-59		20.2%	23.2%	26.2%	29.3%	
60+		20.3%	23.5%	26.7%	29.8%	

FEMALES

AGE	RISKY	EXCELLENT	GOOD	FAIR	POOR	VERY POOR
19-24	<9%	18.9%	22.1%	25.0%	29.6%	>29.6%
25-29		18.9%	22.0%	25.4%	29.8%	
30-34		19.7%	22.7%	26.4%	30.5%	
35-39		21.0%	24.0%	27.7%	31.5%	
40-44		22.6%	25.6%	29.3%	32.8%	
45-49		24.4%	27.3%	30.9%	34.1%	
50-54		26.6%	29.7%	33.1%	36.2%	
55-59		27.4%	30.7%	34.0%	37.3%	
60+		27.6%	31.0%	34.4%	38.0%	

4. *CARDIOVASCULAR TRAINING*

1. We discuss how to burn calories efficiently based on your target heart rate.
2. Interval training is the workout of choice.
    a. Working outside of your comfort zone is key
    b. An excellent type of training for all fitness levels
3. Each profession has a specialized cardio session tailored for each field's own specific needs including the frequency, intensity, and duration of the workouts.
    a. Some jobs are very active already and more challenging physically while others are more sedentary.

NOTE: Check with a physician before attempting these personalized workouts.

4. We state our "Stay Fit Principle": the best way to get in shape is not to get out of shape.

3. *SPORTS*

1. Recommended sporting activities are provided for each profession. We take into account unique time constraints, personalities, activity levels, stress levels, etc. and recommend sports that you will benefit from if you engage in them.
2. We provide different types of aerobic classes that will benefit you.
3. Healthy competition is of great importance.

2. *HOW TO MOVE MORE*

1. Realizing how much you move (or don't move) during the day at work is important. Some professions are very sedentary and work against fitness goals, while others are physically demanding.

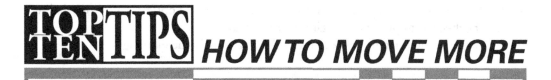

HOW TO MOVE MORE

Estimation of Daily Caloric Expenditure Based on Body Weight and Physical Activity

To calculate your estimated daily caloric expenditure, multiply your body weight in pounds by the calories per pound that corresponds to your activity.

Activity Level	Description	Calories per Pound of Body Weight Expended during a 24-hour period
1	**Very Sedentary** (restrictive movement, such as a patient confined to a house)	13
2	**Sedentary** (most U.S. citizens: light work or office job)	14-15
3	**Moderate Activity** (many college students: some daily activity and weekend recreation)	15
4	**Very Physically Active** (vigorous activity at least 3-4 times/week)	16
5	**Competitive Athlete** (daily activity in high energy sport)	17-19

2.   Your dietary intake determines how you should move more for optimal caloric expenditure.
    a.   High-sugar meals require high intense exercise
    b.   High-fat meals require low & slow cardio first thing in the morning

1. *OBSTACLES & WAYS TO CONQUER THEM*

1.   Every occupation has its own set of obstacles that hold one back from reaching his/her ultimate fitness goals. We state the obstacle and then provide a solution to counteract it.
2.   Our plan makes the "non-obvious" obvious.
3.   Where there is a will, there is a way!

Hot tip: In your professional field, you will see your profession's icon in parentheses with a section of the book next to it. These are the cross references that will help you in achieving SUPER HEALTH. (example.—📖, Calories a person burns daily)

CHAPTER 5

SUPER HEALTH PROGRAMS FOR PROFESSIONS A-L

	<u>Activity Level</u>	<u>Stress Level</u>
	4.0	2.0

1. 55+ & RETIREES ♉

It's part of the job! (♉ all TOP TEN TOOLS)

Let's get the bad news out of the way first. As you are probably aware of, the older we get, the slower our metabolism gets. It slows down at a rate of about 10% each decade after age 35. Therefore, by the time we reach age 55, we will have to work 20% harder than we did when we were 35 and 30% harder at 65 and so on. It's a fact of life that our bodies are imperfect and that over time, the machinery inside will slow down.

Enough with the sour news, getting out of the doldrums into the land of opportunity we see that if you do decide to work harder in the gym and work harder at what you eat, then you can stop this decline in its tracks!

Out of the 300+ clients that we have dealt with, take a guess on who is the best in shape pound for pound. Would you believe it if we told you...

Dick Berkowitz (age 67)
Marvin Lender (age 63)
Murray Lender (age 73)

How can that be you ask? If their bodies are at least 30% weaker than 30-year old men, how can they be in better shape? The answer is quite simple: THEY WORK HARDER and they incorporate the ten tools every day of their lives. If they can do it, I know that you can too! Weight training with challenging resistance is the key. This will keep your muscles so busy that they won't have time to deteriorate. They will be too busy getting stronger. Bones and joints will strengthen along with your heart and mind. Believe me when I tell you that you will be standing more upright with improved posture and gaining greater strength and vigor.

10. *Lifestyle Tips*

Think young, stay active, and lift weights and you will gain all the benefits mentioned above. You will not have to worry about hurting your back from getting up out of a chair. These habits will also help prevent arthritis and combat osteoporosis.

HOT TIP:
#1-

* Rev up that metabolism throughout the day by frequently eating small meals.

Resistance training promotes an independent lifestyle. As a retiree, you will have more time on your hands to do as you please. What better way to spend your leisure time than to hit the waves in Malibu. That's only our opinion. In all honesty, you can have fun outdoors and make your neighbors in Florida envious of you while you mow your lawn with your shirt off or you can set up a nice garden with a tank top and shorts on without a hint of shame. If you are really ambitious, you can get a fun part-time job. This will keep you continuously active and retain a youthful spirit.

9. *All-Star Foods and Liquid Fuel*

Here is a list of top recommended foods to fuel you throughout the day that are low in fat:

cottage cheese	1% milk
legumes	yogurt
wheat pasta	high-fiber cereals (all bran)
chicken soup	mango, citrus fruits*
multi-grain bread products	oatmeal*

*NOTE: Oatmeal (counteracts fatigue)
   Mango, citrus fruits (boosts immunity/slows down aging process)
   Corn
   Spinach & other green leafy veggies (helps prevent damage to skin cells as you age)
   Green tea (boosts metabolic rate)
   Water (50 oz. on a daily basis-vital for skin, muscle, organs, & clearing toxins)
   Asparagus, mushrooms, broccoli, tomatoes
   Grilled chicken breast

Prunes, raisins (high in antioxidants, lowers undesirable cholesterol levels (LDL), raises beneficial cholesterol levels (HDL)

Top round sirloin, ground sirloin (increases testosterone levels in men)

Fish: salmon, shrimp, tuna, cod, mackerel, sardines, crab legs
(reduces the risk of heart disease due to the high amount of omega-3 fatty acids)

HOT TIP:
#1

* When cooking, use flaxseed oil and olive oil.

Here is a list of other foods that help combat the aging process:

Sunflower seeds (highest natural vitamin E content of any food-very important for looking younger)

Yams, sweet potatoes (high in beta-carotene-helps ward off aging wrinkles by the sun's rays)

Grape juice (provides protection from heart attack & stroke, also high in antioxidants which helps the skin maintain a youthful appearance)

High fiber foods (ex. beans) (helps prevent damage to the skin, keeps bones and heart healthy)

8. *Foods to Avoid*

Here is a list of the Top 10 "you will look 80, feel 80, and act 80 foods" to avoid:

1) **Alcohol w/ out moderation** (try to limit your consumption to 2-3 glasses of wine a week w/ your meal)

2) **Fried foods** (ex. fried chicken, French fries)

3) **Foods high in trans fat** (ex. butter, mayonnaise)

4) **Foods high in saturated fat** (ex. whole milk, cheese, corn oil)

5) **Foods high in hydrogenated oil** (ex. margarine, chips, shortening)

6) **Foods high in refined carbohydrates** (fructose-sweetened beverages, soda, white bread (rolls/hamburger buns), potato bread)

NOTE: Low G.I. carbs help avoid type II diabetes.

7) **Rich, creamy entrees** (ex. cheeses on everything-excess calories not needed)

8) **Desserts w/ out moderation** (once a week for indulgence)

9) **Excessive caffeine** (try decaffeinated beverages)

10) **Excessive amounts of chocolate**

HOT TIP:
#1

*If you need a caffeine boost, black coffee with skim milk & sugar substitute is a good alternative to many other high calorie drinks.

7. Meals: How many & when?

On a daily basis, you will most likely not have to deal with the stresses of the working world to the same extent as you once did. Your goal is to help keep your metabolism firing on all cylinders throughout the course of a day.

Eating 5-6 small meals a day every three hours will keep you energized and alert your body to metabolize on a regular basis. This sequence of eating will greatly aid you in defying that 10% decline each decade. Also, this will help stabilize your blood sugar level during the day.

6. Supplementation & Sleep

As we age, it may be difficult getting a consistent sleep throughout the night, but try to get 7 hours with one powernap during the day.

What supplements are right for you?
    A List

    1. multivitamin
    2. antioxidants- help fight free radicals, which are a byproduct of intense exercise and an intense, stressful profession (high in vitamin C & E)
    3. flaxseed oil (pills or liquid form-1000 mg a day)
    4. essential fatty acids (omega 3's)
NOTE: These two oils (3&4) help strengthen thin, brittle hair and keep the skin smooth.

    B List

    1. saw palmetto
    2. glucosamine/chondroitin

HOT TOPIC: *ARTHRITIS*

Over 20 million people suffer from osteoarthritis, which is a degenerative joint disease. This debilitating ailment is often linked to the repetitive use of joints, obesity, joint trauma, and age (wear and tear of joints).
What can be done to reduce the inflammation and pain?

Here is a list of foods and supplements, which can reduce pain & inflammation.

Top 10 Foods & Supplements for Arthritis Sufferers

10. Fruits (especially cherries)
9. Vegetables
8. Whole grains
7. Cold water fish (ex. salmon)
6. Flaxseed oil
5. Omega 3 supplements (fish oil)
4. Vitamin C
3. Glucosamine/Chondroitin**
2. Nuts
1. Legumes

NOTE: This supplement has received much media attention on how it can help arthritis sufferers and those w/ chronic joint pain. They do have a positive effect for some in reducing pain and rebuilding cartilage. Take them as recommended on the bottle and if you feel a benefit within 4-6 months continue to take them, otherwise discontinue the use. **CAUTION: If you are allergic to shellfish, consult your doctor before taking this supplement.

Foods to Avoid

1. Highly-processed snack foods
2. Prepackaged foods
3. Peanut oil, corn oil
4. Cottonseed oil
5. Omega-6 oils

NOTE: These oils are "PRO"-INFLAMMATORY contributing to joint inflammation and pain.

HOT TIPS:
#1

* Strengthen your muscles correctly through resistance training. This will help reduce arthritis flare-ups and improve your flexibility.

#2

* Combine exercising correctly and all-star foods. Focus on strengthening your core muscles such as your abdominal region and your lower back (lumbo-pelvic-hip complex).

#3

* Aqua therapy can also be a soothing, effective relief for your entire body.

5. *Resistance Training*

At around 35 years old, your muscle tone begins to decrease, especially in males as their testosterone levels go down. By age 55, you lose approximately 20% of your muscle tone if you do not engage in a proper resistance-training program. As you well know, a critical factor in having a "kick butt", "firing on all cylinders", more sped up metabolism is having a good amount of muscle tone.

Age? It's only a number to you! So, you young at heart & mind guys and girls, here is a program customized for you:

- 3 days a week
- Total body workouts

     NOTE: Take a day off in between your workout sessions as your body needs a little longer to recover.

Warmup
- 10-15 minutes
- Walk vigorously before hitting the weights to loosen up and get ready for action.
- Perform 50 small arm circles with arms straight out to the side. This will help keep your shoulder joints strong and limber.

BOTH MALES & FEMALES
- 2 sets of each exercise at 8-10 reps
- 70-80% failure for both sets (more advanced can do 80-90%)
- Mix machine training w/ free weight training

YOUR ROUTINE AT THE GYM

25 bodyweight squats (watch your knees, stay back on your heels)

2 sets chest press (machine)

2 sets lat row (machine)

2 sets bicep curls (dumbbells)

2 sets shoulder press (dumbbells)

2 sets leg extensions

2 sets lying leg curls

2 sets supermans (lying on stomach arms extended, raise arms & legs up simultaneously and hold for 3 seconds-15-20 reps)

2 sets (stability ball-if available) crunches (15-20 reps)

HOT TIP:

#1

*If affordable, hire a personal trainer that understands your body. You will be amazed at what you will be able to do!

HOT TOPIC: *KINESTHETIC TRAINING*

Kinesthetic training is defined as knowing where one's body is in space and time.

This will help older individuals avoid simple accidents like falling down or inadvertently missing a step on a stair. Below a list of exercises are included that you can perform "blindfolded" that will help you. These exercises can be done in the comfort of your own home or practically anywhere for that matter.

Stand on one leg and try to balance yourself for a minute.

Walking step over step on a 2x4 on the ground (take it slow).

Perform 15 bodyweight squats.

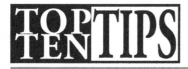

Exercise Helps Reduce Pain

**Percentage of patients reporting a reduction
in back pain after an exercise program.**

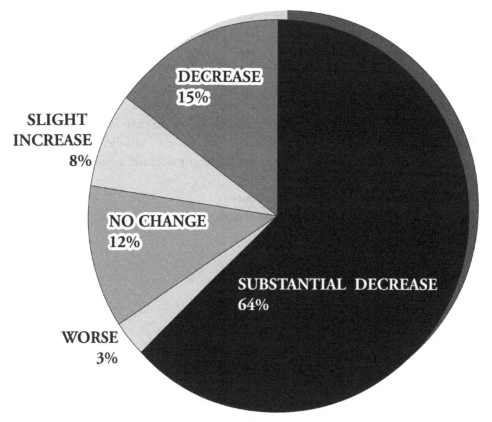

Adapted from- The Clinical Effects of Intensive, Specific Exercise on low Back Pain:
A Controlled Study of 895 Consecutive Patients with 1 year Follow Up,
Nelson et al, Orthopedics, October, 1995

4. *Cardiovascular training* (↟↟ TOP TEN TOPICS, high vs. low intense cardio)

When: 3 days a week after resistance training
How long: 20 minutes (approximately)
Intensity: Intervals

Day 1 (Treadmill)

Time	*Intensity*
8 minutes	walk at 3.8 mph
2 minutes	walk uphill (3.0 incline) at 4.0 mph
6 minutes	walk at 3.8 mph
2 minutes	walk uphill (6.0 incline) at 4.0 mph

Day 2 (Precor elliptical trainer)

Time	*Intensity*
5 minutes	easy & slow
2 minutes	hard & fast
4 minutes	easy & slow
2 minutes	hard & fast
3 minutes	easy & slow
1 minute	hard & fast
3 minutes	easy & slow

Day 3 (Treadmill)

Repeat same times and intensity levels for day 1.

HOT TIP:
#1

* If you do not have a heart rate monitor (ex. polar brand), then go by perceived exertion (PE). Hard and fast should be at a PE of 8 while easy and slow should be a PE of 5.

3. Sports

Enjoy some activities that will get your whole body involved.

- Swimming & aquatic classes
- Yoga & Pilates
- Tennis
- Bocce
- Gardening (220 cal/hr burned)
- Golf (you can burn an extra 320 cal/hr taking a stroll enjoying nature vs. using the cart)

2. How to Move More   Activity level   4.0

Top Tips for Moving More

- Perform the kinesthetic training every other day for about 5 minutes. Those could be some of the best 5 minutes spent.
- Walk whenever and wherever possible. Park farther away from the grocery store and shopping plazas.
- Try to take the stairs whenever it is convenient.
- Buy a walking mower to cut the grass.
- Associate with people that are highly energetic. This will have a positive effect on you and you will have a positive effect on them.
- If you are sitting down, move a body part (ex. foot-in small circles) to keep your muscles active and the blood flowing.

The results of these actions will be outstanding. Your metabolism will be highly active and this will help combat "father time".

HOT TIP:
#1

* Try to keep moving at all times!

1. Obstacles and Ways To Conquer Them

1. Father time   Don't stop exercising or get lethargic as you age. You can fight aging successfully by implementing all of the tools mentioned on a daily basis. You will return to yesteryear and do many of the things you once could do. It's been proven time and time again.

2. Having energy

Incorporate the lifestyle tips, the workout program outlined, and eating the all-star food choices. You will gain an energy unparalleled (possibly outdoing your "30 something" self!). That's exciting!

3. Ailments that may accompany father time

Mentally stay strong and continue to have faith in others and yourself. Staying positive can provide an amazing spark that forces your body to do what the mind says. Stay active. Lift weights. Laugh a little!

Activity Level	Stress Level
1.0	6.0

2. COMPUTER-RELATED ⌨

It's part of the job!

Your job requires a lot of sitting down. Your work requires very little physical sweat (unless you are running late to a meeting or in trouble with your boss!). Working with computers is what you do, so looking at a computer screen for long, extended periods of time is the norm.

Your job may allow you to work out of your home. Late nights on the job may occur from time to time. You may be required to play the part of the hero and "save the system". You may carry a beeper/pager with you often times being on call 24 hours a day (at various times throughout the year) if there is a system malfunction. Being proficient at your job may not be enough. You are an intelligent problem solver, thinking analytically about various options to be had. You are task-oriented in your approach to solving these problems & getting everyone to see your way may sometimes be a modest challenge.

10. *Lifestyle Tips* (⌨ TOP TEN TOOLS, move more)

Move! Move more! Move even more! Get up throughout the course of your workday to stretch or to take a walk or to pick up a memo. Find a reason to get up and MOVE! When you are sitting, sit with good posture. Sit a comfortable distance from the computer. Add a pair of handgrips to your pile of papers & books at your cubicle/desk area to use them for maintaining flexibility in your muscles and joints in your hand.

Due to the sedentary nature of your job, you need to take advantage of every opportunity that your body has to offer. Upon waking up, your metabolism is at its quickest ready to efficiently burn fat molecules. Utilize this time to workout (before work) to rev up your engine early on.

A high priority on your list of "things to do" should be to keep a constant flow of glucose to the brain. Your profession requires a lot of brainpower. Therefore, your blood sugar level needs to be kept constant throughout the day.

9. *All-Star Foods and Liquid Fuel*

FOODS AT WORK

Low glycemic carbohydrates

yams	sweet potatoes
low-fat yogurt	apples
pears	old-fashioned oatmeal

Whole-grained cereals

all-bran cereals   Kashi go-lean
Barbara's shredded spoonfuls   Fiber one

HOT TIP:
#1

*Use the 5/5 rule when buying & eating whole grain cereals. These should have at least 5 grams of fiber and less than 5 grams of sugar.

Other high quality foods

➢ Carrot sticks (helps vision-high in vitamin A), coleslaw, cucumber salad, low-fat cottage cheese
➢ Grilled chicken breast salad w/ olive oil & balsamic vinegar, broccoli, cucumbers, celery, spinach, olives, tomatoes
➢ Prunes (high in antioxidants), avocado, watermelon, papaya, peaches

ALL-STAR SNACKS

➢ Pure protein bars
➢ Luna bars
➢ Clif bars
➢ Pumpkin seeds
➢ Sunflower seeds
➢ Kashi go-lean bars
➢ Trailmix

FOODS AT HOME

➢ Eggs (high in iron), old-fashioned oatmeal, grape juice, grapefruit
➢ Egg-white omelettes w/ kidney beans, veggie cheese, broccoli
➢ Low-fat beef patties (90% fat-free) on multi-grained bread, steamed veggies
➢ Roasted turkey breast, brown rice, zucchini, & mushroom kebobs
➢ Low glycemic meat alternatives: gardenburger, soyburger on wheat pitas
➢ Lean pork tenderloin, red potatoes, asparagus
➢ Good sources of monounsaturated fats:

- Salmon, swordfish, other cold water fish
- Flaxseed oil
- Olive oil

HOT TIP:
#1

*If you can stay strict to this program designed, then you are allowed 1 cheat day a week. Your body's metabolism will be cranking and will subsequently absorb these calories using them for your daily fuel.

Liquid Fuel

- Have water by your desk at all times. A 16 oz. container filled with water is ideal. Fill this up 6 times a day and drink this as opposed to multiple cups of coffee.

8. Foods to Avoid

HIGH GI FOODS

rice cakes	cookies	soda
chips	chocolate	granola bars
bagels	donuts	croissants
muffins	hoagie rolls	nutri-grain bars

CAFFEINE

- ➢ Should be consumed in moderation (if at all)
- ➢ Avoid the caffe lattes, mochas, & light and sweet coffees
- ➢ Stick to black coffee w/ splenda & soymilk

POOR LUNCH/DINNER CHOICES

- Creamy salad dressings on salads
- Double bacon cheeseburgers, French fries, milkshake, apple pie
- Sausage, cheese, pepper grinders
- Fried foods (shrimp, chicken, mozzarella sticks)
- New England clam chowder, clams w/ melted butter
- Eggplant parmigiana, gnocchi's, meatball grinders
- Dark turkey meat, stuffing, pumpkin pie

BAD BREAKFASTS

- 4 sausage links, 3 pancakes w/ maple syrup
- whole milk w/ high sugar cereal
- bacon, egg, sausage on bagels/rolls
- instant oatmeal, hashbrowns

HOT TIP:
#1

*Viewing this list of "Foods to Avoid" should not force you into starving yourself. Eat smaller meals more frequently throughout the day vs. less frequent, more abundant-sized meals to keep that metabolism firing.

7. *Meals: How many & when?*
Five small meals every 3 hours (approx.) is the plan of attack! You must take advantage of all of the tips we put forth for you so you can get your metabolic rate revved up on a consistent basis.

Training Days

*Have ½ meal replacement pre-training followed by the other ½ post-training.

9 A.M.	Small meal
12 P.M.	Small meal
3 P.M.	Small meal
6 P.M.	Small meal
8 P.M.	Small meal

Non-training Days

7 A.M.	Small meal
10 A.M.	Small meal
1 P.M.	Small meal
4 P.M.	Small meal
7 P.M.	Small meal

6. *Supplementation & Sleep*
Get in a habit of obtaining 6-8 hours of sleep daily. Your brain needs sufficient rest for optimal functioning at work the next day. Your eyes need a rest from time to time. Getting away from the computer will save on your eyesight in the long run.

What supplements are right for you?

    <u>A List</u>

    1. multivitamin

    2. antioxidant

    3. flaxseed oil

    4. EFAs

    5. Xenadrine EFX (be careful here-helpful fat burner)

    6. meal replacement

    <u>B List</u>

    1. creatine/glutamine

    2. ginkgo & ginseng

    3. vitamin C

    4. echinacea

5. *Resistance Training*
- Four days: Monday, Tuesday, Thursday, Friday (in the morning)
  - ➢ MONDAY & THURSDAY- Upper body
  - ➢ TUESDAY & FRIDAY- Lower body

A workout right for you!

- 1 hour of circuit training w/ cardio incorporated
- FEMALES: 12-15 reps, 75-85% failure on last 2 reps
- MALES: 8-12 reps; 80-90% failure on last 2 reps

<u>MONDAY/THURSDAY</u> (UPPER BODY)

    ➢ **2 minute rest in between circuits**

    ➢ **15-30 second rest between exercises**

<u>Circuit 1</u>

1)   Chest press machine
2)   Incline hammer strength press
3)   Lat row machine

4) Side lateral raises
5) Dumbbell bicep curls
6) Standing tricep extensions (2 ropes)
7) Seated dumbbell shoulder press
8) Rear deltoid flyes
9) Stability ball abdominal crunches
10) X-trainer elliptical-5 minutes (HR 75-85%)

Circuit 2

- Same 1st 9 exercises in circuit #1.
- Jump rope-5 minutes (rest for 10 second clips if needed)

Circuit 3

- Same 1st 9 exercises in circuit #1 & #2.
- X-trainer elliptical- 5 minutes (HR 60-70%)

TUESDAY/FRIDAY (LOWER BODY)

> ➢ **2 minute rest in between circuits**
> ➢ **15-30 second rest between exercises**

Circuit 1

1) Squats barbell
2) Squat thrusts w/ dumbbells (when you rise up, raise arms over head w/ dumbbells)
3) Lying leg curls
4) Leg extensions
5) Standing calf raises
6) Stationary lunges w/ dumbbells alternating legs
7) Low back extensions machine
8) Jog/run on treadmill- 5 minutes (HR 75-85%)

Circuit 2

- Same 1st 7 exercises in circuit #1.
- Stepmill-5 minutes (HR 80-85%)

<u>Circuit 3</u>

- Same 1st 7 exercises in circuit #1 & #2.
- Jumping jacks- 2 minutes
- Jump rope- 1 minute
- Jumping jacks- 2 minutes
- Jump rope- 1 minute

BENEFITS OF THIS TYPE OF CIRCUIT TRAINING:

- ❖ Your cardiovascular training is included with your resistance training.
- ❖ Your heart rate remains medium to high throughout the circuits so you are constantly burning calories.
- ❖ If done with a challenging intensity, you could easily burn 1000 calories in an hour!
- ❖ It is diverse, not boring.
- ❖ It will be the hardest, yet most beneficial part of the day and serve as that brainpower for later. Problems to solve at work can be accomplished more readily having that extra focus. Things will seem that much easier!
- ❖ Your "EPOC" (excess post-oxygen consumption) will be higher throughout the day resulting in higher calorie burning for 2-15 hours post-exercise. After long periods of sitting, this is just what the doctor ordered!

HOT TIP:
#1

*If you need that kickstart in the morning, go to your local coffee shop and get a small black coffee w/ Splenda.

4. *Cardiovascular training* (⌨ TOP TEN TOPICS, high vs. low intense cardio)
   Good news!
     The 15 minutes of cardio training incorporated into your resistance training is all that you will need. Yes, that's it!

BUT…….
   Do you want to be in the absolute best shape possible?
     Perform 1 hour of low & slow cardio on Wednesday, Saturday, or Sunday morning. Try to maintain your heart rate between 60-65% of maximum throughout the session.

3. *Sports*

Those of you true "computer-geeks" or "gamers", reconsider dedicating all of your leisure time from these computer-related activities like CD games, online games, or interactive gaming to something a bit more rigorous. Enjoy some great stress-relieving outdoor activities.

Enjoy some active, outdoor sports that get the whole body moving.

- Golf (w/out cart)
- Tennis
- Basketball
- Hiking
- Rock climbing
- Swimming
- Softball
- Leisurely outdoor jogs

2. *How to Move More*   <u>Activity level</u>   <u>1.0</u>

We have especially comprised a list of some of the most useful tips for your professional field. Utilize these suggestions below to counteract your low activity level throughout the day. They are "uniquely" unlike any other tips you've seen!

<u>TOP 10 TIPS TO PREVENT "SITTING ON THE JOB"</u>

10. Have a screen saver/alarm clock to alert you that it is time to move.

-Getting up and moving on the hour will keep the metabolism burning.

9. Get up & move around early on in the day.

-At 10 A.M., get up to take a walk outside. Take a nice 10-minute break to breathe in some fresh air. Come back in and take the stairs to your office (if you have stairs). Stretch your hamstrings before sitting down. Touch your toes while keeping legs straight w/ slight bend.

8. Move again an hour later.

-At 11 A.M., get up again. This time do 15 bodyweight squats by your desk.

7. Move again an hour later.

-At 12 P.M., eat your lunch (outside, if possible). Engage in good, stimulating conversation. Tell your friends about your exercise adventure.

6. Move again in 2 hours.

-At 2 P.M., get up out of your seat and do 20 pushups.

5. Move again in an hour.

-At 3 P.M., eat a small meal. Take a walk outside to breathe some fresh air. Clear your mind for a few minutes enjoying the moment.

4. Move again in an hour.

-At 4 P.M., get up and do 15 bodyweight squats.

3. Stay seated this time with good posture.

-Sit with good posture (chest up, abs tight) at all times. Don't stare at the computer all day long. Look away from time to time and give your eyes a break.

2. Move the smaller muscles.

-Use handgrips to help strengthen your hands. This will keep you moving and is an excellent stress reliever. Work the abs each day (15 situps-morning & 15 situps-night).

1. Invest in a stability ball.

-Instead of an office chair, you will burn an extra 200-300 calories a day by using your muscles to help keep you balanced & stabilized. This may seem somewhat strange. Although, at this point, what doesn't sound weird? The point is that you want to have as much control as possible over your well being. Who cares what other people at work think?! You are a leader and on the way to optimal SUPER HEALTH.

*Now, do you understand what we would like you to do??????

1. *Obstacles and Ways To Conquer Them*

1. Sitting down all day	Try to incorporate our Top 10 Tips for moving more into your daily routine at work. Train with that passion & intensity in the morning and you will reap the multitude of benefits that will follow. Set the wheels in motion. That's right, in MOTION! Be a SUPER HEALTH leader by example and you will become the latest and greatest trend in your company!
2. Getting up every morning to train	It's about habits! Don't settle for mediocrity. This is something you must do. Many people who have left a more active profession to sit down in front of a computer all day complain about the loss of energy and gain of girth. Stop this in its tracks! There are no if's, and's, or but's. Our recommended plans will get you into a very healthy and productive routine at work and at home. No more excuses. Your time is NOW!

Activity Level	Stress Level
6.0	3.5

3. DELIVERY DRIVERS & POSTAL 📬

It's part of the job!

Many hours of sitting and driving are required in your professional field. At times, the driving can be an endurance run of sorts, which may be rather stressful. You need to be alert at all times, although that may be challenging (to keep your focus) for long, arduous periods of driving.

Physical labor can be grueling. There may be times of intermittent lifting (possible heavy loads). Work can be monotonous for many of your professions (ex. postal workers-same route, same dropoffs day in and day out) so maintaining an upbeat motivating attitude can be an obstacle to overcome. In today's day and age, everyone depends on you and with the dawning of a high-speed technology-based era (ex. on-line shopping), your job takes on another level of responsibility.

10. *Lifestyle Tips*

TOP 10 TIPS TO "TAKE TO THE STREETS" (& HOME)

10. Always bring your all-star snacks with you to work.
9. Sit tall with good posture while driving.
8. Lift with your legs for heavier boxes/deliveries.
7. Create diversity in other areas of your life (outside of work) to stay well-rounded.
6. Work hard at your job, train harder at the gym, & rest even more.
5. Train at different times during the week (mix it up), depending on your schedule.
4. Keep positively occupied while driving. Listen to motivational tapes rather than letting stressful occurrences on the road (ex. traffic jams, crazy drivers) get the best of you.
3. Eat and train consistently. Control your consumption of coffee throughout the day.
2. While on the road, make a stop and take a break at a peaceful park for lunch (if possible).
1. Above all, you are your own boss! You have to stay self-disciplined in your workouts/diet & remain self-motivated. No one else can give you the strength that you need, but yourself!

9. *All-Star Foods and Liquid Fuel* (📖 all TOP TEN FIT FAST FOODS)

FOODS AT WORK (bring your food with you)

➤ Hard-boiled eggs, Polly-O-string-um lite mozzarella, soy & flaxseed tortilla chips
➤ Peanut butter & jelly on rye, Luna bars, Clif bars, Pure Protein bars
➤ Turkey breast (6 oz.), veggie cheese on multi-grain bread

➢ Box of Grapenuts in vehicle (snack accordingly).
➢ Low-fat yogurt, low-fat cottage cheese, prunes, apples, pears, grapefruits, cherries, kiwi, plums

FOODS AT HOME

➢ Old-fashioned oatmeal, 4 egg whites, grape juice
➢ Salads (make it colorful, mix it up a bit)-use different healthy veggies: olives, asparagus, cauliflower, eggplant, red peppers, green peppers, fat-free cheddar cheese, beets, radishes w/ grilled chicken breast strips, olive oil & vinegar
➢ Brown rice, white roasted turkey breast, corn, peas
➢ Fish (salmon, tuna, swordfish, crab legs)-high in vitamin B, chili, new potatoes
➢ Lean cuts of meat: top round/ sirloin/ flank/ 90% fat-free ground beef/ sweet potatoes, celery sticks, carrot sticks, mushrooms

On the road without all-star foods?

◆ Check out the fit-fast food choices.
◆ Stop at the local supermarket & pick up some healthy choices at the salad bar.
◆ All-natural food stores can provide a great selection of healthy, great tasting, and cost-effective foods for you.

Liquid Fuel

• Caffeine in moderation (1 cup-morning or directly before a workout)
• 16 oz. sports water bottle within arms reach all of the time, fill up w/ water & drink 6 a day
• green tea
• limit alcohol usage (1 cup of red wine every other day)

8. Foods to Avoid

➢ **Foods high in sodium:**
   -frozen food entrees, Chinese food w/ sauces, instant noodles

➢ **Quick hits:**
   -cookies, candy, chocolate, soda, granola bars

➢ **Convenience store foods:**
   -hot dogs, nachos, soda, high-sugar drinks, frozen burritos, chips

➤ **High sugar caffeinated beverages:**
   -caffe lattes, cappuccinos, mochas

➤ **Big meal binges:**
   -pizza, meatball/sausage grinders

➤ **Fried foods:**
   -fried chicken, fried shrimp, French fries, burgers

➤ **Alcoholic beverages:**
   -overconsumption is a problem (limit to 1 cup of red wine every other day)

➤ **Other not so good for you "goodies":**
   -whole milk, high-sugar cereals, sausage, bacon

7. Meals: How many & when?

Your plan here is straightforward. You should ideally consume 5 small meals a day every 3 hours. Try not to eat past 8 P.M. at night if you are a morning riser. What you are consuming is crucial to your overall wellness success. All-star quality carbs & proteins are recommended for each meal. During your training days, consume a meal replacement (drink/bar) directly after you finish your workout.

6. Supplementation & Sleep

Eight hours of sleep is vital for your profession! You need to be alert at all times while driving on the road. You may need to make "X" number of deliveries on a day or you may need to be at a certain location at a specific time. We understand the pressures, but there are rules of the game to obtain SUPER HEALTH state, "For one to be truly effective, one has to be truly awake!" Popping amphetamines, stimulants, and/or power drinks to stay awake are temporary fixes that could have permanent negative effects on your body in the long haul. It is ultimately about your health because that is of HIGHEST priority!

Those delivery rides may be long, boring, and monotonous and as a result, your mind may begin to drift and your eyes may begin to shut. Does this sound familiar? REST, proper rest, is the solution! If you just can't hack 8 hours (for whatever reason) of sleep, try parking your vehicle in a nice, quiet spot/rest area and take a 15-minute power nap to reload from time to time.

What supplements are right for you?
   A List

   1. multivitamin & multimineral
   2. antioxidant
   3. vitamin B (1000 mg)

<u>**B** List</u>

1. ZMA
2. melatonin
3. tyrosine
4. ginkgo & ginseng

5. *Resistance Training* (📖 TOP TEN TOPICS, proper form)

- Three days a week (48 hours of rest in between workouts)
- 1 day-morning/1-day-lunch time/1-day-evening
- Perform this workout for 3 months, then try "Best Workout That You've Never Done"-topic #4

A workout right for you!

<u>DAY 1</u> High repetition workout

- FEMALES & MALES : 75% failure on last 2 reps
- 1 minute rest between sets

    1)   25 pushups
    2)   25 squats
    3)   15 standing dumbbell military presses (use manageable weight)
    4)   Walking lunges (no weight-perform for 1 min. in open space in gym)
    5)   Pull ups (as many as you can for 2 sets-use assisted machine if necessary)
    6)   15 seated leg curls (use manageable weight)
    7)   15 lying leg curls
    8)   15 dips (use assisted machine if necessary)
    9)   75 crunches (split into 3 sets)

<u>DAY 2</u> Free-weight workout

FEMALES: 3 sets/exercise, 12-15 reps; 75-85% failure on last 2 reps
MALES: 3 sets/exercise, 8-10 reps; 85-90% failure on last 2 reps

    1)   Dumbbell bench press
    2)   Barbell squats
    3)   Dumbbell bicep curls

4) Weighted step ups (18 inch bench)
5) Dumbbell side raises
6) Dumbbell stationary lunges
7) Lying dumbbell tricep extensions
8) Hanging leg raises w/ medicine ball between ankles

DAY 3 Machine workout

FEMALES: 3 sets/exercise, 12-15 reps, 85-95% failure on last 2 reps
MALES: 3 sets/exercise, 8-10 reps; 90-99% failure on last 2 reps
    NOTE: It is easier and safer to go to failure using machines rather than free weights.

1) Seated leg press
2) Seated leg extensions
3) Standing calf raises
4) Incline hammer strength chest press
5) Seated lat rows
6) Standing tricep extensions on cables w/ 2 ropes
7) Preacher curl machine
8) Low back extension machine
9) Abdominal crunch machine

HOT BODY PARTS
$$$ LOW BACK $$$

Incorporate low back extensions (lying supermans) into your nightly routine. Each night before bed, perform 20 supermans (with both arms and legs held out for 3 seconds above the ground).

$$$ SHOULDERS & ARMS $$$
These body parts must be strong for the type of work that you perform. Train them with passion and they will respond when you ask them to in the future.

4. *Cardiovascular training*
    ❑ **3 days a week, 15-20 minutes after resistance training**
    ❑ **diversify your workouts**

DAY 1

- 5 minutes on stationary bike (HR 70-75%)
- 5 minutes on step mill (HR 75-80%)
- 5 minutes on x-trainer (HR 80-90%)

DAY 2

- 5 minutes- jump rope (stop for 15 seconds if you can't do 5 minutes)
- 5 minutes run/jog- incline treadmill (3.0) (HR 85-90%)
- 5 minutes x-trainer elliptical (HR 85-90%)

DAY 3

- 15 minute interval training on mode of choice

TIME	INTENSITY	HR
3 min	slow & easy	60%
3 min	fast & hard	80%
3 min	slow & easy	65%
3 min	fast & hard	85%
3 min	moderate	75%
5 min	cool down	55%

3. *Sports*
Enjoy some active, outdoor activities.

- hiking
- mountain biking
- rock climbing
- cross-country skiing
- kayaking
- ice skating

If you are an indoor person, challenge yourself!

- ❖ cardio kick-boxing
- ❖ Yoga
- ❖ spinning
- ❖ Pilates

Get your competitive juices flowing.

- softball
- deck hockey
- recreation (league) basketball

2. How to Move More <u>Activity level</u>   <u>6.0</u>

There are times when you are driving and sitting for long, extended periods of time. With this very sedentary state comes the other part of your job. Your activity level rises when you make your deliveries. You may have to move, lift, push, or carry various items short or long distances. Here are some recommended tips for driving, sitting, and lifting.

Driving:

Be certain to check your posture. Keep your chest up, shoulders back, and your abdominals tight (drawing your belly button in to your spine while driving). It is easy to let yourself slouch in your seat for long periods of time. Purchase a cushion that you can situate in the lumbar region of your back. This will be very beneficial for some of those longer trips. Have a pair of handgrips by your seat to help reduce tension.

If you are driving for longer than an hour, it would be a good idea to stop at a rest stop and stretch your hamstrings by touching your toes and holding for 15 seconds. Also, some body squats with your arms hoisted high above your head and your fingers pointed at the sky would help maintain flexibility in joints and muscles. This will preserve the muscles in your lower back and help maintain postural alignment and stabilize your inner and outer core units.

Lifting & Moving:

Lift from the bottom up! Lift with your legs, arms, & shoulders as opposed to your lower back. Don't lift too many boxes at once in an attempt to save time. One bad move and you will be spending time in physical therapy.

Do not put yourself in precarious positions. Carrying boxes over your head or having to bend down and reach for something out of range can be compromising and cause a twist/tear of the muscle. Compound that with adverse weather conditions and things can get even more treacherous.

If you have many deliveries to make, do not rush! This will just add further undue stress to the day & you may find yourself distracted while driving.

HOT TIP
#1

*Postal employees: Try to walk your mail door to door as much as possible (provided the environment is safe). This is excellent exercise for your body. Carry some pepper spray with you to avert any would be predators if need be.

1. *Obstacles and Ways To Conquer Them*

1. Falling asleep or becoming groggy while driving

If you are driving long periods, it is important to have your all-star foods with you at all times. You may want to pull over to the side of the road and breathe in some fresh air to recuperate. If you are falling asleep at the wheel, pull over to take a powernap and then drink some water to hydrate yourself.

2. Boredom from driving/loss of driving focus

It is all about being self-motivated. We can advise you to stay focused, but that's easier said than done. Listen to some motivational tapes. These tapes are critical key success factors for people. Following voices and absorbing their advice will force you to listen to them. Watch the coffee drinking. If you are a habitual daily drinker, then you will have to drink more coffee to have the same effect.

3. Training intense after a tough day at work

Take a 10 minute powernap right after work. Then, you can consume that medium black coffee (right before a workout). This will get you fired up and ready for an outstanding workout.

4. You are depended on & expected to, but recognized & appreciated?

Remember that you hold a very important position! Set your standards high for yourself at work, at the gym, & with your eating habits. A great work ethic will either sooner or later gain its notoriety by your co-workers & bosses. Word of mouth is one of the most powerful resources & you will be received with great ambition.

5. Staying motivated in the gym

As we've mentioned, mix up your workouts and have fun. Bring your headphones and listen to your favorite, most stimulating workout music. Train with a friend and make it a point to go together at set times.

	Activity Level	Stress Level
	4.0	5.5

4. EDUCATION ✎

It's part of the job!

Let the show begin! You are often times putting on a show 5 times a day, 5 days a week, 180 days a year with live performances. You impact the lives of many on a daily basis with your actions of what you say, as well as what you do. To grasp the attention of your audience, you need to have charisma and be a leader. Being a good public speaker is a demanding, yet rewarding task. To be effective in what you do, you must possess qualities of good character including honesty, fairness, responsibility, trustworthiness, etc. The vacations are what make it great! As you say, the three best things about your profession are June, July, & August!

10. *Lifestyle Tips*

Bring your food with you to work. Many times, the faculty and staff will be "rewarded" with goodies brought in from the outside and you will deviate from healthy eating. Have your all-star selected foods by your side at your desk or working area so you don't have to venture to the faculty lounge for a quick splurge. You can maintain a stable blood sugar level throughout the day with good eating habits. This will help in keeping the same energy and vigor that you had in the morning for later in the day.

Workout early in the morning, if possible. Otherwise, hit the gym after work for a solid session. You have the time to dedicate; therefore, keep it consistent with your schedule of working out 3 days during the week and once on the weekend. You will look better and feel better. Managing children and/or other adults effectively takes sufficient energy. Often times, the complaint of many educators is a feeling of burnout. Keep your body energized by getting the consistent 8 hours of sleep each night. Properly fuel your body with good foods and follow a workout plan that is right for you.

During those stressful days, take a timeout. Get away from work, take a break through a fun activity and clear your mind. Take advantage of your time off to regroup mentally. The summertime can be used as a great opportunity for challenging yourself physically and attempting new recipes for success that will enhance your overall health wellness.

9. *All-Star Foods and Liquid Fuel*

FOODS AT WORK

- meal replacements, Pure Protein bars, Clif bars, Luna bars, Balance bars
- apples, pears, peaches, blueberries, strawberries, grapes
- multi-grained bread w/ turkey breast, carrot sticks
- canned albacore tuna on pumpernickel bread w/ hot sauce & veggie cheese
- low-fat yogurt, Progresso soups, rye crackers w/ hummus, coleslaw

FOODS AT HOME

- lean beef (sirloin, top round, tenderloin pork), sweet potato, sautéed spinach w/ red pepper, mushrooms, olive oil
- cobb salad (avocados, tomatoes, hard-boiled eggs, low-fat blue cheese, chicken, bacon bits)
- salmon, swordfish, mackerel, shrimp, sushi—BRAIN FOOD high in iodine, vitamin B and omega 3 fatty acids
- beans (soy, pinto, lima, kidney), grilled chicken breast, brown rice
- oatmeal, egg whites, grapefruit/orange juice (morning)

Liquid Fuel

- WATER (100 oz. daily)-have 20 oz. by your desk and constantly fill it up
- GREEN TEA-contains antioxidants helping to offset the accumulated stresses throughout the day

HOT TIP:
#1

*Portion your meals. You want to be conscious of the amount of food consumed per sitting. Even an excess caloric intake of the selected all-star foods results in unwanted weight gain. Here are portion sizes that you are recommended NOT to exceed.

Visual Cue	Approximate Size	Food Choices
Baseball	1 Cup	Medium piece of fruit/ Baked or sweet potato
Rounded Handful	½ cup, 1 oz.	Rice, cooked veggies
Cassette Tape	4 oz.	Meat & poultry
Checkbook	4 oz.	Fish

8. Foods to Avoid (✎ all TOP TEN RESULTS)

Not eating throughout the day can be much worse than eating the following avoided foods:
LACK OF FOOD=LACK OF SUSTAINED ENERGY=LACK OF PRODUCTIVITY AT WORK & AT THE GYM

That is a double no no!!

Quick reminder: You are what you eat! You can feel like it, smell like it, and may even look like it!

➢ chips, cookies, soda, candy, high-sugar cereals, chocolate, vending machine foods & other quick hits
➢ pizza/other greasy foods from the cafeteria lunch
➢ high-carbohydrate drinks (especially during the day and before training)
➢ too many caffeinated beverages (limit to 1 a day)
➢ trans-fat foods (margarine, fried foods w/ corn oil)
➢ sausage, bacon, pancakes

7. Meals: How many & when?

The idea here is to get in 4-6 small meals a day to keep the motor running smoothly and evenly efficient throughout the course of a workday. During the week through Saturday, stay disciplined to your diet and workouts. On Sunday, live it up and reward yourself with your most desired foods. Then, get back on the "Road to SUPER HEALTH" train for Monday-Saturday. The focus for your meals is that you eat frequently rather than going for too long without food. If you do not eat small frequent meals throughout the day, your body will not know when its next meal is coming and will store it as fat for survival.

*Morning workout

6 A.M.	½ meal replacement & fruit
6:30 A.M.	workout session
7:30 A.M.	½ meal replacement
9 A.M.	breakfast (1st meal)
12 P.M.	lunch
3 P.M.	snack
6 P.M.	dinner

*Nighttime workout

6-7 A.M.	breakfast
10 A.M.	mid-morning snack
1 P.M.	lunch
3 P.M.	mid-afternoon snack
5 P.M.	workout session
6:30 P.M.	meal replacement
7:30 P.M.	dinner

*Non-training days

7 A.M.	breakfast
10 A.M.	snack
1 P.M.	lunch
4 P.M.	snack
7 P.M.	dinner

* Schedule may be different for each profession, but sequence and intervals are the same.

6. *Supplementation & Sleep*

The recommended 8 hours a day is vital towards your overall wellness throughout the day and giving your audience a 100% virtuoso performance everyday. Can you make up for lost sleep during the week on the weekends? No, you can not! Making up sleep on the weekends should be a hint to you that you are losing needed sleep during the week. Dedicating 1/3 of your life to sleeping will greatly enhance the other 2/3 of your life.

MYTH: As you get older, you don't require as many hours of daily sleep.

FACT: Everyone needs at least 8 hours of sleep a night for optimal functioning.

What supplements are right for you?

<u>A List</u>

1. multivitamin & mineral
2. vitamin B (100 mg)
3. EFAs
4. glutamine

<u>B List</u>

1. tyrosine
2. melatonin

5. *Resistance Training*

Three days: Monday, Wednesday, Friday (morning or evening)
Duration: 40-45 minutes

MONDAY *(total body blitz-3 total circuits)*

➢ MEN=8-10 reps/set (80-85% failure last 2 reps of each exercise),
   WOMEN=12-15 reps/set (70%-75% failure on last 2,3 reps)
➢ Maintain heart rate at 60%
➢ No rest in between exercises within the circuit

NOTE: If you are ambitious to get in tip-top shape, perform the Monday workout highlighted below once more on the weekend.

A workout right for you!

Circuit #1

1) 50 body squats to warm-up
2) Dumbbell chest press
3) Lying leg curl
4) Lying skull crushers (two dumbbells)
5) Machine shoulder press
6) Leg press
7) Lat pulldowns
8) Low back extensions
9) Leg raises (hip thrusts, lying on back)

REST FOR TWO MINUTES

Circuit #2

Repeat circuit #1 and rest for two minutes.

Circuit #3

Repeat circuit #1/#2.

WEDNESDAY *(upper body)*

➢ MEN=8-10 reps/set (80-90% failure),
   WOMEN=12-15 reps/set (75%-85% failure)
   3 sets per each exercise
➢ 1 minute rest in between exercises and sets

1) 50 arm circles to the front and rear
2) Flat bench press
3) Dumbbell incline press
4) Lat rows
5) Preacher curls
6) Standing tricep extensions
7) Side raises
8) Dumbbell shoulder presses
9) Hanging leg raises

FRIDAY (lower body)

➢ MEN=8-10 reps/set (80-90% failure),
   WOMEN=12-15 reps/set (75%-85% failure)
   3 sets per exercise
➢ 1 minute rest in between exercises and sets

1) Squats
2) Lunges (stationary, alternate legs)
3) Seated leg curls
4) Seated calf raises
5) Wall squat (hold as long as you can)
6) Stability ball crunches

FACT: By age 25, if we stop working out, we lose muscle and metabolic speed.

4. *Cardiovascular training* (✎ TOP TEN TOPICS, high vs. low intense cardio)

After you have completed resistance training for the day (Mon/Wed/Fri), perform 15-20 minutes of fairly intense aerobic training. Go at your own speed, but try and push yourself a little more each time. The elliptical x-trainer is highly recommended as an outstanding mode of cardio for its ability to utilize most muscles in your body. It has sensors on the handles that read your heart rate. This piece of equipment is low-impact, meaning that it doesn't put a lot of stress on your joints and ligaments.

Here is a selected workout for a 40 yr. old person. (adjust your own heart rate)

	Max HR=180
Time	**Heart rate**
3 minutes	140
2 minutes	150

3 minutes	140
2 minutes	155
3 minutes	145
2 minutes	160
5 minute (cool down)	<140

3. *Sports*

For most education professions, you have the luxury of having the summers off. This allows you to spend time outdoors and enjoy the weather while you get some exercise playing your favorite sport (ex. basketball, golf, swimming, etc.).

As a coach, you may have access to a gymnasium and be able to set up some friendly games to play. If you are coaching or decide to coach a team, then you could get those competitive juices flowing which will give you more energy, enthusiasm, excitement, and fulfillment in life.

You may also need a mental recharging during the course of the school year with all of the hustle and bustle throughout each day. Escaping to a peaceful, serene place could be your answer.

This well deserved time off can also provide you with the ability to try some extreme sports or challenging physical events that you normally wouldn't try during the school year. If your goal is to become excellent at a sport, then you can do it with the means that you have. Fortunately, you have time to achieve your goals with a good discipline and mental frame of mind.

Try some "not so run of the mill" sporting activities
- Triathlon
- Biathlon
- Decathlon
- Mountain biking
- Kayaking
- Hiking
- Yoga/Tai Chi
- Karate
- Bodybuilding
- Road races

2. *How to Move More*   Activity level   4.0

You are most likely standing throughout a good portion of the day. Make sure that you stand with good posture, shoulders back, head straight up, and chest up.

"Keep the performance going" tips

- Take the stairs everywhere.
- On your breaks/periods off, walk the halls or go outside to get some fresh air.
- If you have access to a gym at your place, go there for a while to shoot some hoops.
- During the summer, get a side job where you can do something you enjoy while you get exercise (ex. paint jobs, building jobs, sports instructor/coach, etc.)

1. *Obstacles and Ways To Conquer Them*

1. Resting 8 hours a night

Stay disciplined each night during the week and obtain 8 hours of sleep. Go to bed the same time each night and your body will have no problem waking up at the same time. You will be able to sleep naturally each night and have the energy that can match or even better your students. Use your off time during the day for planning and grading. Don't procrastinate and wait until night time to start.

2. Becoming complacent and lazy during your time off.

Focus on a fun, invigorating activity, coaching a youth's sports team, or engaging in a sport or some physical activity that will really get you going each day. Set some goals to achieve during the summertime. This will also give you a better focus throughout the school year.

3. Getting all of your meals in

Bring your all-star foods with you everyday. Have them in close proximity at all times. This will reduce the temptation for "quick fixes" or skipping a meal during the day.

<u>Activity Level</u>   <u>Stress Level</u>
4.5   7.5

5. HEALTHCARE

It's part of the job!

You are involved in the well being of our society. You are responsible for saving people's lives and attempting to rid the world of pestilence. Without your vast expertise in an all-important medical profession, many of our loved ones today may not exist and experience a quality life. Without your tireless efforts, often times round the clock, we would not have such rapid advances in medical technology and extend our time on this planet.

You need a strong-willed mentality complemented by a soothing, caring heart in dealing with patients and their families. You are patient, a good listener, an unselfish helping hand, compassionate and cool under pressure. In a high stress environment, you have to keep a smile on as a sense of assurance for different situations that may arise.

As a healthcare professional, you spend a good deal of your life exercising your mind. Your sleep may be disrupted, at times, with a life-threatening emergency at any time of the day. Your days may even be long so your energy levels need to be as high as possible for conducting sound health-conscious decisions.

Burning calories at work may not be a problem for most of you by moving all day from one place to another. You may not burn the same amount of calories that a manual laborer will by lifting heavy objects and performing physically exhausting activities. Although, you are on your feet quite often moving around, which will enhance the fat-burning process (burning calories-80% of the time).

10. *Lifestyle Tips*

Rest, train, and work hard! You may enjoy the rich things in life, but watch what you feed your belly. Limit your alcohol consumption. Instead of power lunches, participate in power workouts.

Encourage exercise and sound eating to all of your patients/co-workers. You are an important figure in the community so your words and actions will carry weight. You are a role model and should lead the way toward a healthier path. Your body requires proper fuel at the proper times. Bring your all-star foods with you to work so you won't have to resort to ingesting any "quick hits" to keep you going.

Set weekly goals for yourself in relation to your overall wellness. We recommend for you to develop a contract with yourself for achievement. Set up an "I WILL" chart with your weekly goals and track your progress. Here is an example:

I WILL.........

1)   **work out 4 times this week**
2)   **sweat at the end of each workout**

3)   devote my entire focus into working out
4)   eat my all-star foods on a consistent basis

NAME: _____ DATE: _____

WEEKLY COMMENTS (below):

Track your weekly successes and see what you have accomplished. As the weeks progress, you will be astounded by your accomplishments and will gain a sense of pride about what you can do and will continue to do. Remember, in order to help others achieve wellness, you need to help yourself first. Exercise is one of the finest outlets possible for relieving stress and experiencing a natural euphoric state while getting that much closer to SUPER HEALTH. If you can afford to hire a personal trainer, then do so. It can certainly be to your benefit to work with someone who can motivate you to workout regularly. The two of you will sit down and discuss some fitness goals and how to attain them. You will feel more dedicated to the goal as you are tracked for your progress each visit.

9. All-Star Foods and Liquid Fuel

FOODS AT WORK

- ➤ **Citrus fruits:** grapefruits, oranges-help boost immunity
- ➤ Apples, pears, prunes, blueberries, cherries, strawberries, raisins
- ➤ Berries-help prevent menstrual cramping & varicose vein formation in females; packed with nutrients that help prevent different diseases
- ➤ Clif bars, Luna bars, Kashi Go-Lean bars, low-fat yogurt, cottage cheese
- ➤ Grilled chicken breast on pumpernickel bread, tomato & onion salad
- ➤ Sushi, dried lentils, three-bean soup
- ➤ Sliced turkey breast (4 oz.) on rye crisp bread, coleslaw, deli pickle

Eating out?
- ➤ Minestrone soup with out the cheese
- ➤ Pasta (2 handfuls) with tomato sauce, no cheese
- ➤ Pizza with veggie toppings (half or no cheese)

FOODS AT HOME

- ➤ High-fiber breakfast cereal (All-Bran, Fiberone, Barbara's Shredded Spoonfuls, Grapenuts, Total), 4 eggwhites, grapejuice (12 oz.)

- ➢ Grilled chicken breast strips on iceberg lettuce, broccoli, cucumbers, peppers, tomatoes w/ low-fat balsamic vinegar dressing
- ➢ Top round sirloin, sweet potato, corn on the cob
- ➢ Veggie burger, whole wheat spaghetti, grilled asparagus strips
- ➢ Fish (salmon, tuna, shrimp, swordfish; baked/broiled)-helps your body counter stressful situations, w/ cracked barley, legumes & steamed veggies

Liquid Fuel

- Water (100 oz. a day)
- Caffeine-free herbal teas (green tea)
- Soymilk
- Fruit$_2$O

HOT TIP:
#1

*Cook w/ olive oil. It is an essential fatty acid that is important for healthy skin, nails, and helps in lowering the threat of heart disease and colon cancer. Flax oil is also a good alternative for cooking.

#2

*Use hot sauce on some foods. Studies show that capsaicin, which is the main ingredient in jalapeno peppers, can boost your metabolism up to 20%. You will burn more calories for up to 3 hours after your meal.

8. Foods to Avoid

Foods high in trans fat (the new killer)

margarine	non-dairy creamers
French fries	frozen entrees
processed vegetable fat	pre-made dips
processed packaged foods	dry gravy, sauce mixes

HOT TIP
#1

*Check your food labels (ingredients section) for the words "partially hydrogenated" or "hydrogenated vegetable oil". This indicates that the food product contains commercially synthesized trans fat. Soon all foods will disclose trans-fat on the labels and it will be easier to avoid these "hidden killers".

Foods high in saturated fat

fatty cuts of meat, pork, bacon, sausage	nachos
whole milk	creamed vegetables
double cheeseburger	desserts

Saturated fat has more of a "storage effect" than monounsaturated fats like olive oil and flax oil. Monounsaturated fats are used more readily for energy while saturated fats can clog your arteries increasing your risk for cardiovascular disease. Foods high in saturated fat also contribute to a "lower thermic effect", which ultimately lowers your metabolism.

Foods high in sugar

granola bars	candy	cookies
chocolate	soda	ice cream
graham crackers	donuts	mashed potatoes
jellybeans	French bread	waffles w/ blueberry topping

Other foods to avoid

➢ Grinders (white hoagie rolls) w/ cheese, mayonnaise, fried chicken
➢ Alcohol (limit the intake)
➢ Caffeine (limit the intake-cut back to one cup a day if you are a caffeine junkie); avoid lattes, mochas, light & sweet coffee
➢ Appetizers during cocktail hour or before dinner (dips, chips, cheeses)
➢ High-fat salad dressings
➢ Instant oatmeal

7. Meals: How many & when? (🔲 TOP TEN TOPICS, glycemic index)

Breakfast is the most important meal of the day for you. It is extremely important if you set your sights on the gym that day. We realize that your schedule may be quite busy and that you can get so consumed in work that breakfast may be your only meal for 12 hours until late at night. We want to adjust the eating schedule just a bit. Eating right is a big priority in your life or at least it should be. It should come FIRST!

Private practice?

After breakfast, eat small meals every 3 hours consisting of small carb/moderate protein/low fat. This will provide you with a steady stream of energy throughout the day to keep energy levels high and fat metabolism in full operation. You may be helping and saving people's lives all day long and you don't often know when during the course of the day you will experience a life-threatening emergency that will require your complete focus.

On call? Odd hour shifts?

Breakfast is still of paramount importance. Also, eat a solid lunch during the day with moderate carbs/protein/fat and have a smaller dinner reducing the carb/fat intake and increasing the protein uptake. Between meals, enjoy some all-star snack choices. Try not to eat within 2 hours of going to sleep.

6. Supplementation & Sleep

Sleep may be something that you haven't gotten much of in the past. It may be erratic, broken up, or even lacking, especially if you are on-call as a doctor or an EMT.

Try to average 6-7 hours of sleep a night if you don't have a private practice, otherwise 7-8 hours is recommended for private practice physicians. If need be, try to make up for some missed sleep during the day by taking a powernap. You must rest to be alert for the people that you treat daily. They are putting their faith into your hands for sound, wise decisions that will help them. If you work different shifts, try to get to bed the same time everyday and develop consistent sleeping patterns.

What supplements are right for you?

<u>A List</u>

1. multivitamin
2. antioxidant
3. EFAs
4. vitamin C (1000 mg)
5. melatonin

<u>**B** List</u>

1. echinacea
2. vitamin B (100 mg)
3. glutamine (10 g)
4. calcium
5. ginkgo & ginseng

5. *Resistance Training*

Three days a week preferably at lunchtime will be a good time for you to perform your workouts. Lunchtime workouts break up the day nicely. This is a good time to clear your mind and relieve some built up stress. Your glycogen levels should be full due to a couple of good meals consumed earlier on.

HOT TIP
#1

*Track your progress in the gym by keeping a journal of your goals & accomplishments.

A workout right for you!

<u>DAY 1 </u>(Total Body Blitz)

- Beneficial for those faced with high-pressure and intense situations at work
- Challenging for your body physically which helps when you are challenged mentally
- Exercises performed back-to-back with 30-60 seconds rest in between

    1) wall squats (iron chair)-hold for 1 minute
    2) chinups (palms facing you)-12-15 reps
    3) dips (keep chest up, don't let upper arms go below parallel to the ground)-15-20 reps
    4) squat thrusts (take 15-20 lb. dumbbells (males) 5-10 lb. dumbbells (females)-hold to side and squat down, rise up, explode, thrust dumbbells over head using shoulders)-15-20 reps
    5) treadmill run (get heart rate up to 80-85%)-2 minutes
    6) rest for 2-3 minutes
    7) perform same circuit
    8) rest for 2-3 minutes
    9) perform same circuit

HOT TIP
#1

*Go at your own fitness level, but whatever that level may be, challenge yourself and try to get to the next level each workout.

<u>DAY 2</u> (Upper Body Blast)

- FEMALES: 3 sets, 12-15 reps, 75-85% failure on last 2 reps
- MALES: 3 sets, 8-12 reps, 80-90% failure on last 2 reps
- Train with free weights to create an unstable, challenging environment recruiting more muscle fibers to action

  1) Warm up w/ 50 arm circles to the front & rear
  2) Dumbbell chest press
  3) Seated lat row
  4) Seated dumbbell curls
  5) Side lateral raises
  6) Lying dumbbell tricep extensions
  7) Abdominal crunches on stability ball
  8) Low back extensions on 45 degree bench
  9) 50 pushups

<u>DAY 3</u> (Low Body Destruction)

- Repetition scheme the same as above for day 2 exercises

  1) 50 body weight squats
  2) leg press
  3) 25 jump squats
  4) lying leg curls
  5) 50 jump ropes
  6) leg extensions
  7) 75 jumping jacks
  8) standing calf raises
  9) hanging leg raises

Ambitious?

- ❖ Do a 4th day of resistance training using the "Total Body Blitz" workout again!

4. *Cardiovascular training*
- ❑ **3 days a week**
- ❑ **Set weekly goals**

DAY 1

- After your total body blitz workout has been completed, shift gears to run a mile either on the treadmill or on a local track. Set goals to beat your last time.

DAY 2

- Ride the stationary bike or walk for 1 hour first thing in the morning w/ out eating breakfast (HR 60-65%, low & slow).
- Pick the easiest morning of the week.
- This will burn a great amount of fat.
- This will aid in mental alertness at work throughout the day.

DAY 3

- For 15 minutes after your leg workout (preferably)

Use the x-trainer elliptical incorporating your legs & upper body to raise the heart rate more rapidly.

TIME	INTERVAL	HEART RATE	*LEVEL
3 min	low & slow	60-70%	8
2 min	fast & hard	80-85%	12
2 min	low & slow	65-70%	9
2 min	fast & hard	80-85%	13
1 min	medium	65-75%	10
2 min	fast & hard	80-90%	14
1 min	medium	65-75%	10
2 min	fast & hard	85-90%	15
5 min	cool down	60-65%	5

*Adjust the levels manually increasing/decreasing your level intensity.

3. *Sports* (📖 TOP TEN TOPICS, Yoga & Pilates)
Enjoy some get away from the crowd activities

- **Golf**- take a walk and enjoy the scenery & a friendly round of competition
- **Hiking**- get those leg muscles working and enjoy a great escape being close to nature by yourself or w/ that special someone

HOT TIP:
#1

*Attach a backpack with 10 lbs. on your back for a challenging climb. Wait and see how great you feel when you've reached the top of the mountain.

- **Yoga & Pilates**- These are gaining popularity in becoming the 21st century "stressbusters". There are various instructors in your region. This is not just for females any longer. All types, all ages can benefit.

2. *How to Move More*   <u>Activity level</u>   <u>4.5</u>

<u>Private practices</u>

➤ Sit with good posture.
➤ Take the stairs in office building.
➤ In between clients (or every hour), do 10 sky-to-floor squats. Stand, squat down, touch floor w/ fingers, stand up & stretch hands towards the sky.

<u>On feet, moving a lot</u>

➤ Take the stairs in hospital or office building. When this becomes routine, take 2 stairs at a time.
➤ Wear comfortable shoes that will support your lower back.
➤ Perform 15 squats before lunch.
➤ Keep good posture while performing duties (surgeries).

1. *Obstacles and Ways To Conquer Them*

1. Finding time to workout   You spent long hours working for your professional certification in the healthcare industry. As a healthcare worker, you realize the priority that exercise should take in your life. Set weekly goals and record them in a journal. Hold yourself accountable and

write down any reasons for skipped workouts or cheated meals. You will have a better handle on efficient time management and what you, personally, need to do to obtain your goals.

2. Devoting all of your positive energy and focus into your clients/ patients and having enough energy for then a workout

Your health is the #1 priority in your life. If you fall ill on a frequent basis or you are not at full capacity, you are of limited use to the people surrounding you. Working out will help strengthen your immune system and rebuild your mental focus for the day. You are a respected figure in the community. Lead by example and pave the way to a healthier life style.

3. Remaining positive around negative circumstances

You put on many caps during the course of the day. You are a health-care worker, a counselor, a decision maker, a duty performer, a family man (woman) to name a few. Don't forget to take care of yourself first. Enjoy your time with your family. Spend time doing different activities, going on special trips, participating in your child's activities. Take good care of your body by eating well & exercising frequently.

4. Excessive alcohol consumption to help you relax

Keep it all in moderation. We realize the severe implications that alcohol can have on both you and others that you are associated with. These alcoholic beverages are empty, low nutritive value calories. Alcohol is a depressant drug that can deprive you of alertness, focus, concentration, and coordination. All are key factors for a successful day at work.

5. Setting challenges

Uphold the standard that you set for yourself and others. Your strong mind will allow you to achieve anything that it wants. Take your flare and passion that you bring to work and use it in the gym. You are a role model whether you like it or not. A little more pressure to hit the gym consistently, eat right, and get proper sleep may be just the right prescription that the doctor ordered!

Activity Level	Stress Level
5.5	7.0

6. HIGH PROFILE $

It's part of the job!

You are in the public eye daily, weekly, yearly, for that matter, ALL OF THE TIME! The pressure is on to look good and impress those that you are "selling yourself" to or communicating with. You possess a powerful presence with more incentive and motivation to stay fit. Your high energetic, charismatic personalities keep everyone attracted to what you are doing. Your work schedule may fluctuate day-to-day or week-to-week. For models and actors, your body is your meal ticket. Taking good care of it is a main priority. We understand the value of portraying a good image to the public.

10. *Lifestyle Tips*

Working out will be a tremendous benefit in many ways. You need to look good and keep that youthful glow on your face, so physical activity will be of the utmost benefit. Having a personal trainer can suit you well to reach physical fitness goals easier. They are specialized experts in the field of health and fitness that can help you focus on your time in the gym, not letting distractions get in the way. The "crazy" hours that you may work are often times an excuse for not working out. A personal trainer will set some goals for you to attain and will be there for you to rely on and keep you moving forward climbing the wellness ladder.

Your diet is extremely important, not just for your overall appearance, but for your overall sustained energy level throughout the day. You can not afford to be sick because opportunities/jobs may come up that require travel and you have to be there ready to go. Media personnel may be required frequently to travel to various sites. If you are sitting for extended periods at work going over newscasts, etc. then keep your abdominals tight, as strong abs lead to a strong low back.

Plan ahead to put some allotted time aside for family, friends, and working out. This will keep you balanced as best as possible. Watch your food intake and moderate your stress levels. As being in the limelight, you promote the lifestyle that you practice and live on a daily basis. Often times, there seems to be an abundant supply of food available on sets or at conferences. Make wise decisions to when and what you consume. You are a role model for many whether you'd like to be or not. You are a leader and looked up to. Portraying the right message can be a very powerful tool to have in your arsenal.

As a politician, your health leads to more votes. Having a youthful appearance and that vim vigor will set you up for success. Our recent presidential leaders, such as Bill Clinton & George W. Bush, have set the standard for living complete lives and performing better at work by consistently incorporating exercise into their daily routines.

As a model/actor, you may be compelled to go on strict diets to lose a lot of weight quickly or (for a specific role) put on a lot of weight rapidly. This will hurt your overall well being and lifestyle if this becomes a consistent habit in your life. Keep in mind that the goal is towards SUPER HEALTH, long-term overall wellness (physically & mentally).

9. *All-Star Foods and Liquid Fuel* ($ TOP TEN TOPICS, low carb/high protein diets)

FOODS AT WORK

➢ **Restaurants**: order smaller portions, grilled/broiled choices of quality protein (ex. grilled chicken breast, brown rice, sauteed spinach & pepper in olive oil)
➢ **Cruciferous veggies**: carrots (aids in healthy skin), green leafy veggies, broccoli, asparagus
➢ Tuna sushi, California rolls, fresh steamed veggies, miso soup
➢ Citrus fruits, mangoes, low-fat yogurt, cottage cheese (high in calcium-good for bones, teeth & muscle)
➢ Albacore tuna fish on rye bread w/ lettuce & tomato, three-bean salad

FOODS AT HOME

➢ **Complex carbohydrates**: oats, yams, sweet potatoes (helps keep skin strong & high in vitamin A + antioxidants-help slow aging process), barleys, beans
➢ Eggs (high in iron), veggie burgers, tofu, veggie cheese, soymilk, low-fat milk
➢ Lean red meat (ex. top round sirloin, flank steak), whole wheat pasta, cucumber salad
➢ Chicken soup, red potatoes, roasted turkey breast w/ hot sauce, fruit salad
➢ **Good fat sources (excellent for the skin)**: fish (salmon, swordfish, mackerel, orange roughy – stabilizes the heart), olive oil, flaxseed oil (high in valuable monounsaturated fats)

Liquid Fuel

• Consume 100 oz. water daily. If you travel frequently, drink approx. 40-50 oz. more to keep hydrated.
• Green tea- (enhances metabolism)

8. *Foods to Avoid*

➢ **Alcohol, social drinking**
  • 12 oz. beer has 150 calories
  • excessive alcohol has many detriments, one being that it will gradually affect the appearance of your face and body causing a bloated look
  • limit 1-2 glasses of wine weekly

- ➢ **At restaurants**
  - Creamy entrees, creamy salad dressings
  - Appetizers/desserts
  - Caffeinated beverages
  - Pancakes w/ blueberry topping
  - Sausage, egg, cheese muffin
  - Big pasta entrees (high, dense calories: one bowl can be easy to eat and also easy to tack on over 1000 calories for the day)
- ➢ **Foods high in trans-fat (affects your appearance)**
  - Fried snacks & food (potato chips, corn chips, fried chicken, fried mozzarella sticks, fried zucchini)
  - Crackers
  - Pre-made dips
  - Packaged instant noodles
  - Dry gravy, sauce mixes
  - Cake mixes
  - Processed packaged puddings
  - Whipped dessert toppings
  - Non-dairy creamers
- ➢ **Frozen food entrees**
  - High in sodium, trans-fat
- ➢ **High GI carbs (make you feel bloated)**
  - Bagels
  - Hamburger rolls
  - Hoagie rolls
  - White rice
  - Rice cakes
  - High-sugar cereals (more than 5 grams of sugar)
- ➢ **Luncheon meats**
  - High in sodium

HOT TIP:
#1

*Actor and models: Don't deprive yourself of eating and develop poor eating habits. Many who have come before you have suffered the sad effects of anorexia/bulimia. Also, you don't have to succumb to societal pressures of drinking to have fun or escape life's trials and tribulations. We provide SUPER HEALTH tips to get you on the right track.

7. Meals: How many & when?

Your schedule may be jam packed with places to go and people to meet. You may not have complete control over what it is that you get your hands on to eat and when. Therefore, you may not be able to eat frequent small meals based on your on-the-go schedule. The good news is that you have total control of what you actually get your hands on and put into your body while you are on the move. If there is a will, there certainly is a way!

The general rule for you high profilers is to EAT DOWNHILL! Eat smaller meals every 3-4 hours after breakfast. Upon waking up should be your biggest meal in terms of calories. Each meal following should contain a good proportion of high quality carbohydrates (low GI carbs) and protein. This will give you a long-lasting steady source of energy throughout the day.

Try not to eat past 8 P.M. (even if you are working the 11:00 P.M. news). You will not feel the push to feed the beast if you have properly tamed it throughout the day. Stay disciplined to the best of your ability and remember that someone out there is always working harder than you.

6. Supplementation & Sleep

Rest is vital towards overall wellness. Looking good and being super healthy may be grave challenges ahead if you decide to skip getting that all-important rest. It will creep up on you like a bed bug late at night and turn you from what was once "the consummate professional" into a "has been of the past". We are not intending for this to sound depressing. We just want you looking your best and on the road towards SUPER HEALTH! A consistent 7-8 hours will do the trick. Even a 10-15 minute power nap in a quiet place during the day will restart your engine.

3 MAJOR COMPONENTS TO *SUPER HEALTH*:

1)   **EAT HEALTHY**
2)   **EXERCISE REGULARLY & CORRECTLY**
3)   **GET PROPER REST**

❖   Leaving out #3 above from the equation for SUPER HEALTH will negate #1 & #2.

In showbiz, you will be attending many functions that are most likely scheduled for later in the evening. Plan your schedule so you can obtain at least 7 hours of sleep for that night. Actors, models, and musicians, manage your schedules to meet at more appropriate times than late at night for rehearsals and practices. The motto "Life is one big party" can be true if you exercise and eat well consistently AND if you get the proper rest consistently.

What supplements are right for you?
A List

1. multivitamin
2. meal replacements
3. antioxidants (slows aging, reduces wrinkles, destroys free radicals)
4. EFAs

B List

1. saw palmetto (males)
2. ginkgo, ginseng, tyrosine
3. melatonin

5. *Resistance Training*

2 WORDS: short, intense
WHEN: 3 days a week:
DURATION: 45 minutes

ROUTINE: push, pull, legs

- If you can afford to, put a quality gym into your home
- Workout incognito (can use a personal trainer) to clear your mind
- Find out when you have a consistent free hour where your energy level is highest (morning (ideal), afternoon, evening)

Note: The important thing to realize is that this workout will give you that cutting edge over the competition. You will feel ready to perform more readily and be more productive in front of the camera (or whatever audience it may be)

Workouts during the workweek:
- As an example, train Monday, Wednesday, Friday

A workout right for you!

- FEMALES: 3 sets/exercise, 12-15 reps, 75-85% failure on last 2 reps
- MALES: 3 sets/exercise, 8-10 reps; 80-90% failure on last 2 reps

<u>DAY 1</u> Push (exercises that push away from your body)

Warm up-50 small arm circles to front & rear

1) Dumbbell incline presses
2) Side lateral raises
3) Standing tricep extensions (2 ropes)
4) Machine chest press
5) Dumbbell shoulder press
6) Rear delt flyes

<u>DAY 2</u> Pull (exercises that pull towards your body)

Warm up-50 small arm circles to front & rear

1) Seated lat rows
2) Seated dumbbell curls
3) Seated lat pulldowns
4) Seated preacher curl
5) Low back extensions
   a. machine
      or
   b. 45 deg. torso bench holding circular weight on your chest

<u>DAY 3</u> Legs

Warm up-50 bodyweight squats

1) squats/leg press (if you haven't developed good form w/ squats, try leg press)
2) 100 jump ropes (1 set)
3) Lying leg curls
4) Leg extensions
5) 100 jumping jacks (1 set)
6) step ups (alternate legs on 18 inch box)
7) 50 jump ropes (1 set)
8) 50 jumping jacks (1 set)

HOT TIP:
#1

* Every night before you go to sleep, do 50 crunches lying on the floor. Go slow while controlling your breathing and form.

4. *Cardiovascular training*
- 3 days a week of mind-clearing cardio is a big stress reliever for 15-20 minutes after resistance training
- Always leave each cardio session having broken a sweat

If you like to jog:

- Jog with proper form
- Heel to toe, heel to toe
- Keep your head and chest up

For the ambitious-minded athlete in you:

- 1 day a week (in addition to your 3 days of cardio), perform a 30-minute bout of cardio first thing in the morning before you eat anything.

3. *Sports*
Enjoy some fun activities that will allow you to get away from everything

- golf (walk and enjoy nature)
- hiking
- mountain biking
- skiing
- ice skating
- kayaking
- fishing

Find out which activities you truly enjoy and that relax you. If you have a passion to excel at a specific sport, make time to engage in it to get better. Never be afraid to ask for personal advice from specialized experts in that field.

2. How to Move More   <u>Activity level</u>   <u>5.5</u>

At times, you may be traveling. Sit with good posture. Keep your mind stimulated and drink plenty of water. This will actually force you to go to the bathroom.

There may be a lot of "down time" waiting for shoots or preparing for performances. Again, sit with good posture, stay focused, and even fidget. Stand up and stretch from time to time. Take in a nice deep breath and stretch for the sky and exhale while touching your toes holding for 10-15 seconds steady.

Just in case you didn't hear it the first or even the second time, sit and stand with **good posture** (chest up, spine erect, shoulders back). Your 6'0 frame can look 5'9 or 6'3 depending on how you take care to maintain good posture. Your posture also tells people what you feel about yourself. Good posture displays an air of confidence that can affect your ability to book that job as an actor or model. You are powerful and you want this power to be displayed.

You always want to make a good first impression to your audience. As a politician, you are meeting all kinds of people and your body language can work for or against you. A strong powerful handshake is always a sign of confidence. Keep handgrips by your desk or while traveling from place to place. These not only strengthen your grip, but also reduce built-up tension.

Some days when you are less active, make it a goal of yours to perform 100 bodyweight squats spread out throughout the day.

1. Obstacles and Ways To Conquer Them

1. Always in the public eye	You have to be on all the time! This can become tough at times. Like anything else, it is a job-a limelight job nonetheless. Enjoy your time alone w/ family & friends. Develop good habits & take part in the activities you enjoy that benefit your overall wellness. Exercise is the best prescription for unwanted tension and stress!
2. Eating well around "not-so-well for you" tasty foods	Control your cravings. Keep breath mints r sugarless gum in your opocket. Don't live in the typical "party-zone" that often provides excesses of NON-all-star food choices. Take a moment to give yourself a lifestyle check to the people in your profession and where you are now and where you want to be in the near future!
3. Developing a consistent, productive workout routine	3-5 hours dedicated to resistance & cardio training out of an available 112 hours awake during the week is really not asking much. A "little" self-discipline spent towards obtaining wellness

will give you that much MORE time on this planet, feeling like the star that you are. This will go a long way towards your successes at work.

4. You must always look "good", sound "good", smile "good", , act "good" speak "good"

Is that enough being "goods"? Talk and about daily pressures. You are under a microscope much of the time. Many people may look for you to fail or even relish in it. Here is the solution for all of that toxicity. Don't take yourself so seriously. Remember, you are a human being. Many people would love to be working in your field now. Be proud of your accomplishments. Avoid excessive alcohol consumption and foods high in sugar and trans fat. Do you remember the equation to reach SUPER HEALTH?

Exercise well + eat well + sleep well = (**SUPERHEALTH**)

	Activity Level	Stress Level
	5.5	8.5

7. HIGH RESPONSIBILITY DECISION MAKERS ☻

It's part of the job!

Does this remind you of anything: high anxiety, stress, responsibility, decision making, long hours? Oh, that's right, your JOB! You are dealing with people on a daily basis. You are a problem solver, a mediator, a take action kind of person. You possess leadership qualities and good people skills that attribute to your controlling, take charge nature.

Time is money as they say in business. Your long hours at work may include sitting for prolonged durations. How is your energy level throughout the day? You may wonder, "When will I find time to eat throughout the day?" Often times eating out at social functions or business luncheons may be your meals throughout the day. Lunch may be at noon one day while the next day it is at 2:30 P.M. You may not bring a lunch because you simply don't have enough time in the day to sit down, relax, and eat.

10. *Lifestyle Tips*

Exercise is of utmost importance! It will help ease your mind, allow you to think more clearly, and get rid of built-up tension and stress accumulated throughout the day. It serves as a good escape AWAY FROM WORK. If possible, train before work, as this will set your mindset up for a successful day. Also, your body will be a more efficient calorie-burning machine throughout the day. You may find yourself getting bogged down with last second "projects" that need to be completed and you will not have the energy to complete a solid workout after work. Working out early, speeds up your metabolic rate for the remainder of a potentially long day.

Know your personality!

CEOs, VPs, GMs:
> With the amount of hours that you put in on a daily basis, having enough energy is vital for your physical and mental wellness. Looking and feeling healthy physically, mentally, and emotionally are important, as this will also set the example for the rest of the company.

WALL STREET:
> Dealing with the ups and downs each day can wear on you. Be cool though! Don't get overzealous when a business deal goes well or a stock you purchased doubles in value. Reciprocally, don't go for the nearest bar to drown your sorrows when a stock plummets or a deal goes awry. You do not need to add insult to injury. Both eustress (stress over a pleasant event) and especially distress (stress over an unpleasant event) can be diabolic if not catabolic. Stress can lead to a breakdown of tissue not conducive to lean muscle growth.

The key to your (often times) stressful days is to comprise a list of coping methods that you will utilize in various situations. You can then accompany your personalized formulated plan with a customized workout plan provided.

When you are not working, do exactly that! Because of the demanding stress level, it is very important that you leave your work at work. For obtaining what we call "SUPER HEALTH", you need to understand that you have a life outside of work that is valuable. Enjoy time with your family, engage in a favorite activity, chat with a friend or family member on the telephone. DO NOT WORRY YOUR LIFE AWAY!

When you are on the road or at business luncheons/dinners, you must discipline yourself with correct eating habits. These habits involve eating the "All-Star Foods" that we recommend.

Encourage your staff to become more health conscious. You are a leader in more ways than you know. You set the example. Your staff can experience all of the great benefits from working out. They will have more energy to perform, be more positive-minded, be more goal-oriented (in many ways), work harder, which will ultimately result in greater achievement and more productivity. Be an inspiration! This is the true quality of you as a leader.

9. All-Star Foods and Liquid Fuel

FOODS AT WORK

Here is a list of top foods to fuel you throughout the day.

LOW GLYCEMIC CARBOHYDRATES

brown rice
legumes
pumpernickel/rye bread
apples/pears

QUALITY LEAN SOURCES OF PROTEIN

chicken breast
smoked turkey breast
tuna fish

Liquid Fuel

water-16 oz. sports bottle
(fill up 5 times a day & drink)

green tea (good source of caffeine)
skim milk/soy milk

SNACKS

cottage cheese	**low-fat yogurt**
Pure Protein bars	**Luna bars**
sunflower seeds	**pumpkin seeds**

FOODS AT RESTAURANTS

Two delicious meals that would satisfy:

1) Grilled chicken breast, baked potato, steamed veggies

OR

2) Spicy halibut roll, tuna sushi, salmon sushi

NOTE: Always order foods that are broiled, grilled, poached, or steamed.

FOODS AT HOME

fish (reduces the risk of heart disease due to presence of omega 3
fatty acids)
whole grain cereals (5/5 rule-at least 5 grams of fiber & less than 5 grams
of sugar)
egg whites, oatmeal, juice (orange, apple, cranberry)-for breakfast
lean beef (ex. top round sirloin, flank steak-delivers oxygen to cells &
keeps them energized)
salads w/ fibrous, nutrient dense veggies(ex. broccoli, spinach, carrots,
cauliflower, peas, tomatoes)-include olive oil & balsamic vinegar

HOT TIP:
#1

*Take 2 hours during the weekend to grill your chicken breast and prepare your other foods for the
upcoming work week.

8. *Foods to Avoid*

A) <u>At the restaurant for lunches/business meetings</u>

fried foods	**dessert**
creamy dressings	**alcohol** (limit to 1 drink or none)
appetizers	**deli sandwiches**

B) <u>Fast food restaurants /quick lunchtime takeouts/processed foods</u>

NOTE: Those 2 hours preparing your food on the weekend will save you $$$ & time. Your abs will be sure to thank you later!

C) <u>White flour foods</u>

bagels	**white bread**
rolls & buns	**white rice**
pasta	

D) <u>Whole-milk cheeses</u>

Cheddar, Swiss, Jack

E) <u>Condiments</u>

butter, mayonnaise

F) <u>Quick hits</u>

candy, cookies, chocolate, soda, cake

7. *Meals: How many & when?*

Eat every 3-4 hours with more carbohydrates in the morning time and less throughout the rest of the day.

Monday, Wednesday, Friday (workout days)-when you work out, have half of a meal replacement (high in protein) shake w/ fruit a half an hour before the workout and drink the rest after the workout. Then, eat breakfast within one hour (post-training). Breakfast should be your largest meal of the day w/ the most carbohydrates consumed early on. This meal is vital for providing sustained energy required for optimal performance at work. If you have to get up an hour earlier than normal, do it. Your physique will thank you later. For the rest of the day, divide your meals to be eaten every 3-4 hours with less emphasis on foods containing carbs after 5 P.M.

Tuesday, Thursday, Saturday (non-workout days)-The biggest meal of the day is still in the morning accompanied by smaller, frequent meals every 3-4 hours. Do not go very long without eating. Your body will think that you have suddenly escaped the high intensity of work to a deserted island in every sense of the word. Your body will go from a state of anabolism (building lean muscle mass) to a state of catabolism (breaking down lean muscle mass). In 6 hours time, your body is put in a perfect state to release cortisol (a primary catabolic hormone secreted in response to physical stress). This is not good! Your hard earned muscle will begin to slowly waste away. Your body experiences a feeling comparable to when the Dow Jones drops 300 points drastically or an important client decides to get up and take his/her business to your competitor. Your body needs something that it once had that made it strong. You get the idea!

Sunday-Think of this day as a "reward day" rather than a "cheat day". You are allowed to indulge this day for your wonderful discipline exhibited throughout the week. Your body and mind will be prepared to come back strong for another good week. After all, you are only human even though you are expected to perform at levels far superior. Only allow yourself this cheat day if you have stayed the course from Monday thru Saturday.

6. Supplementation & Sleep

You must get 7-8 hours of sleep a night consistently or you will be setting yourself up for failure. You must develop consistent sleep patterns for mental and physical conditioning. The nights before you work-out, you may consider getting to sleep earlier to rise early for the next morning's workout.

What supplements are right for you?
    <u>A List</u>

1. multivitamin
2. antioxidants- help fight free radicals, which are a byproduct of intense exercise and an intense, stressful profession (high in vitamin C & E)
3. meal replacement
4. EFAs

    <u>B List</u>

1. caffeine before training (100-200 mg)
2. tyrosine

3. B-complex (1000 mg)
4. melatonin

HOT TIPS:
#1

* Caffeine taken 15 minutes right before a workout will provide that kickstart first thing in the morning and give you a great workout.

#2

* Do not get into a habit of drinking caffeinated beverages throughout the day. Your body will soon adapt and it won't have that same igniting effect for which it was intended.

5. *Resistance Training*

This customized workout program is specific for your activity level (5.5) and stress level (8.5). Again, your goal is to get in three solid days of training. Ideally, weekdays of Monday, Wednesday, and Friday in the morning would be optimal. This will get you started on the right foot with the right mind set, setting you up for success at work. Distractions are minimal at this time of the day, also. Warm up for 5-10 minutes with a steady walk or a slow jog. The following workout will take under an hour to complete. Your successes will be multifold for the rest of the day.

A workout right for you!

- 3 days a week
- Each day-circuit training w/ cardio mixed in.
- GUYS: 10-12 repetitions
- GIRLS: 12-15 repetitions
- 75% failure on last rep.

CIRCUIT #1

1) Machine chest press
2) Seated lat rows
3) Dumbbell bicep curls
4) Machine shoulder press
5) Leg press
6) Leg curls (lying)
7) Leg extension
8) Stability ball crunches
9) 100 jumping jacks

NOTE: The key here is to move from exercise to exercise with minimal/no rest. The reason being is to keep your heart rate at 60% max throughout. Rest for 3 minutes before beginning the next circuit.

CIRCUIT #2

- Same resistance training as circuit #1.
- 3 minute run on treadmill (med-hard-70-80% max h.r.)
- rest for 2 minutes

CIRCUIT #3

- Same resistance training as #1/#2
- 5 minutes on stepmill (med-hard-70-80% max h.r.)
- 5 minutes on treadmill (walk/slow jog cool down)
- Stretch

HOT BODY PARTS
$$$ Low back $$$

*Perform 20 repetitions of supermans each night before you go to sleep. Raise your legs and arms up simultaneously and hold for 3 seconds.

4. *Cardiovascular training*

Follow the outlined cardio program incorporated in resistance training. If you are the ambitious type (which I know many of you are!)....

- Take one morning (either Tuesday or Thursday) & do 45 min.-1 hour of cardio first thing in the morning. You can jog, walk uphill (incline) or pedal on the bicycle low and slow (H.R. 60-65%)

3. *Sports*

Looking for a friendly game/activity or that competitive outlet?

- Organize a company softball team (helps build better rapport)
- Road races
- Mountain biking
- Golf (enjoy nature's beauties, compete with yourself & others)
- Tennis (great competitive sport-provided your knees are intact)

2. How to Move More   <u>Activity level</u>   <u>5.5</u> (✪ all TOP TEN TOOLS-especially #9, move more)

Top Tips for Moving More

- Sitting at your desk all day? Have an alarm or a beeper alert you on the hour to MOVE. This may sound silly, but unless you are notified of this, you may get caught up for an indefinite period of inactivity.
  - ➢ Every hour, perform one of the following exercises:
    1) 15 body squats with good form
    2) 15 pushups
    3) Keep legs straight w/ slight bend in knees & bend down, touch toes, stretching hamstrings. Hold steady for 15 seconds.
- When seated, sit with good posture (shoulders back, chest up).
- Try to take the stairs whenever it is convenient.
- When traveling by way of a plane, train, or automobile, sit w/ good posture and drink plenty of water.
- Have handgrips by your desk. This strengthens hands, relieves built-up tension throughout the day & keeps you moving.

1. *Obstacles and Ways To Conquer Them*

1. Time

Actually, this will not be an obstacle if you are disciplined and put your health and well-being as a priority. Plan your workouts in your schedule and value them as much as you would an important business meeting. Hold yourself accountable! Three times a week for an hour a day will make the other 16-17 waking hours that much more productive.

You wouldn't be where you are today, holding this important position, if you didn't take pride in your work and put forth a great deal of passion, intensity, and challenges. Take this same mental approach to the gym & the rest will take care of itself.

CEOS/GMS

2. Running a successful business and leading good employees

You set the example! Actions speak louder than words in the long run. If you exercise regularly, eat well & implement this as a major quality, then your employees will see this and begin to examine their own well being. Put a gym in the office building and serve many healthy choices in the cafeteria. You will be pleasantly surprised at the real power that you truly possess.

WALL STREET
  3. Burning out

When away from work, don't work. By implementing your workouts & all-star foods into your schedule weekly & getting the appropriate amount of daily rest, your energy level will soar up to days of the past.

	Activity Level	Stress Level
	6.5	5.0

8. HOTEL & RESTAURANT ☯

It's part of the job!

You are dealing with people on a daily basis. Often times, you are in a fast-paced environment where customer satisfaction is of the utmost importance. Your customer service and people skills go a long way in how effective you are in your position. You may be on your feet for extended periods of time without a break during busy hours. Lifting, moving, and standing are action verbs often associated with your occupation. Many of you are surrounded by food, possibly even in a hot, steamy environment, during the day.

10. *Lifestyle Tips*

It's a simple equation! Eat well + train well + rest well = looking well + acting well + feeling well = getting paid well (physically, mentally and literally on the job!) It is correct that the equation is simple; although, there are quite a few variables to contend with here. The challenge of being around food 90% of the time (ex. wait staff/bartenders) may make things a bit challenging. You have some choices to make. If you eat where you work, choose healthy all-star food choices. Make note of when you eat. Do not pick and graze all throughout the day. Control your cravings by having healthy snacks from the all-star food list that we provide by your station at work. As a cook, you understand the ingredients that go into various foods; therefore you are a fountain of knowledge when it comes to eating well. Keep a smile on at work and stand/walk with good posture (chest up/shoulders back). To provide that necessary energy to sustain you throughout those long (often times double shifts) days, you will reap the benefits from your all-star food choices and a good customized workout program (best performed prior to your shift).

9. *All-Star Foods and Liquid Fuel*

FOODS AT WORK

Here is a list of quick snacks (meals) if you can not take a break:

> **pure protein bars**
> **apples/pears/strawberries**
> **carrots/soynuts/Brazil nuts/almonds**
> **sunflower seeds**
> **dried apples/dried apricots/dried pears**
> **Luna bars/Clif bars**

QUALITY LEAN SOURCES OF PROTEIN

chicken soup
low-fat yogurt
tuna & salmon sushi
cottage cheese
low-fat milk
ground sirloin

On your lunch break:
sliced turkey breast w/ 1 slice low-fat cheese on
pumpernickel bread (optional-lettuce & tomato)

If you have time to sit down to eat a meal:
Cobb Salad: avocado, tomato, chicken breast, hard-boiled
eggs over lettuce
Large tossed salads: mushrooms, iceberg, cucumbers,
olive oil, celery, vinegar, shrimp

Liquid Fuel

Keep a gallon of water with you and consume ¾ of it daily.

FOODS AT HOME

egg whites, oatmeal, orange juice, grapefruit
90% fat-free patties lean meat/veggie burgers, veggie cheese,
barley products
baked potato, grilled chicken breast, steamed veggies,
baked beans
eggplants, roasted asparagus, yellow squash, corn on the cob
cold-water fish, wheat spaghetti, kidney beans

HOT TIP:
#1

*CAFFEINE

Limit to 1 cup a day (if needed). Your activity level is fairly high throughout the day and you want to stay hydrated. Caffeine is a stimulant and is a diuretic that causes a release of water from the body. You have to drink two 12 oz. cups of water to make up for drinking one 12 oz. cup of caffeinated coffee.

8. *Foods to Avoid* (❂ TOP TEN TOPICS, glycemic index)

This may in fact be your most important tip to follow. You are around fresh, out of the oven, off the stove aromas that are pleasant to the pallet. These fatty foods can lure you into a foreboding place of indulgence. Again, you have choices to make. The correct choice for these particular situations is to STAY DISCIPLINED!

A) High-sugar foods

chocolate	mashed potatoes
cornflakes	instant oatmeal
granola bars	apple pies

B) High-fat foods

whole milk	whole milk cheeses
butter	mayonnaise
French fries	fried mozzarella sticks
fried chicken	macaroni & cheese
chicken pot pies	

C) Liquid killers

alcohol	soda
high-sugar fruit drinks	caffeinated lattes/
	mochas/light & sweet
a pot of coffee daily	

D) High amount of pastries/desserts

croissants	scones
cookies	ice cream
donuts	muffins

E) Rich & creamy entrees

eggplant parmigiana	chicken parmigiana
ravioli	chicken salad w/ Caesar dressing
creamed vegetables	burger w/ cheese

HOT TIP:

#1

*Be careful of any bread or whole-grain product that has enriched flour as its primary ingredient. These foods have high G.I. levels.

7. Meals: How many & when?

#1 Most important meal of the day=BREAKFAST

You have a long day ahead of you. Your busy day will keep you moving, burning calories consistently. This meal will get your metabolism kick-started for the day.

#2 Important meal of the day= 1 hour after working out

Your workout should be performed prior to your shift. In order for this meal to count and do its job properly, you should have a meal replacement shake directly following training to reabsorb lost nutrients. For you, it's all about keeping your energy levels high early on to fuel you accordingly throughout the day.

#3 Eat small, frequent meals every 4 hours or so

Feed the machine frequently! Your activity level is above average so these meals are essential to your success. This is a major reason why keeping your all-star snacks by your station or in close proximity will serve you well. Most likely, there will be stints during the week where you don't get a chance to take breaks for 4-5 hours at a time. With all-star snacks in close quarters, you will keep your metabolism cranking all day long and there won't be any more of these late night binges. After 8 P.M. you will not have the sudden urge to gorge on a less than all-star quality meal.

Here's the breakdown:	*Training days
1. Breakfast-biggest meal	8 A.M.
2. Workout (11 A.M.)-eat meal replacement	12 P.M.
3. Lunch-2nd biggest meal	1-2 P.M.
4. Small meal or all-star food	4 P.M.
5. Small meal or all-star snack	7 P.M.

	*Non-training days
1. Breakfast-biggest meal	8 A.M.
2. Small meal	11 P.M.
3. Small meal	2 P.M.
4. Small meal	5 P.M.
5. Small meal	7 P.M.

* Schedule may be different for each profession, but sequence and intervals are the same.

6. *Supplementation & Sleep*

It is critical that you obtain 7-8 hours of sleep on a daily basis. Waiters, waitresses, and bartenders are very active and always on stage, so rest is vital. Often times, you will feel like crashing when you get home. Sometimes, the scheduling could throw off your sleep patterns if you have to close and then open the following morning. Get as much sleep as possible and thereafter, get back on track. Get that much needed sleep for optimal performance.

What supplements are right for you?

A List

1. multivitamin
2. antioxidants-help fight free radicals, which are a byproduct of intense exercise and an intense, stressful profession (high in vitamin C & E)
3. meal replacement
4. EFAs

B List

1. vitamin B (1000 mg)
2. tyrosine

5. *Resistance Training*

This customized workout program will help keep a positive mind frame throughout the course of a day. Your program will incorporate the use of free weights to help strengthen muscles and improve balance.

A workout right for you!

- 4 days a week

- Short, intense workouts
- Split routine
- Workout every other day (day of rest in between workouts)
- GUYS: 8-10 repetitions; 3 sets; *80-90% failure on last 2-3 reps
- GIRLS: 12-15 repetitions; 3 sets; *70-80% failure on last 3-4 reps

*Fitness level dependent-if you are at a higher level of conditioning, you can push to a higher % failure maintaining proper form.

Day 1-Legs

2) Squats
   - best to perform due to constant standing all day
   - help to improve posture in your upper body
   - recruit major muscles of the legs
3) Step ups (18-inch box)- hold 2 dumbbells to your side(should challenge you)
4) Lying leg curl
5) Standing calf raises
6) Hanging leg raises-works abdominal region

Day 2-Chest & Triceps

1) Dumbbell flat bench chest press
2) Incline dumbbell flyes
3) Lying dumbbell extensions (a.k.a. skull crushers)
4) Standing tricep extensions
5) 100 pushups

Day 3-Back & Biceps

1) Pull ups (use assisted machine if needed)
2) Seated lat rows
3) Seated dumbbell bicep curls
4) Seated preacher curls
5) Low back extensions (45 deg. bench)

HOT BODY PARTS
$$$ Shoulders & Abs $$$

Day 4-Shoulders & Abdominals

1) Dumbbell shoulder presses

2) Seated lateral (side) raises
3) Seated rear deltoid flyes
4) 100 arm circles to front and rear
5) Stability ball crunches
6) Lying leg raises

4. *Cardiovascular training*

Throughout the day, your activity level is already high (6.5) so be careful here. You can easily run yourself thin and burn out if you overdue it. You are on your feet the majority of the day and your body requires sufficient energy in order to be successful.

A plan for sculpting your body:

- 3 days a week after resistance training
- 15 minutes cardio (post-training)
- use different modes each time
  (ex. stationary bike/stairmaster/elliptical x-trainer)
- 3 minutes (even, steady pace-65-70%)
- 2 minutes (harder pace-75-80%)
- Alternate 3 min/2 min intervals for 15 minutes

HOT TIP:
#1

*Wear good supporting shoes, especially while at work.

3. *Sports* (❧ TOP TEN TOPICS, Yoga & Pilates)

- Spinning classes (gives you a chance to get off of your feet for a while and enjoy an intense choice of cardio-burns approx. 600-800 calories per session)
- Mountain biking
- Swimming
- Yoga & Pilates
- Cross-country skiing/downhill skiing

2. *How to Move More*   Activity level   6.5

At work, you are most likely moving adequately throughout the day. Be sure to follow the top tips outlined and further movement will not be required.

Helpful daily tips to keep in mind

- Wear good, comfortable shoes that support your feet. You will be on them for most of the day.
- Always maintain good posture.
- Lift and transfer items at your job using your legs, arms, & shoulders rather than your lower back.
- Stretch every 1-2 hours (bend over, legs straight w/ slight bend in knees, touch toes and hold for 15 seconds for a good hamstring & lower back stretch)

1. *Obstacles and Ways To Conquer Them*

1.Around food all day long

Bring your all-star snacks and food choices with you daily. Refrain from temptation of those great tasting, high-fat, high calorie foods that you are around. Remember to have your highest calorie meal at breakfast & eat smaller meals throughout the day. Don't pick between meals and after 8 P.M. your food factory should close.

2. Standing all day

Develop a habit to stand with good posture and train with good posture. Remember the habit rule! It takes 21 days to create a habit, good or bad. Let's make them good!

3. Getting plenty of rest

Stay disciplined to the **best** of your ability. Your "best" does not include after-work parties on a daily basis. That may or may not get tiring after a while, but for certain your body will not have the energy to workout, which is a necessary component for SUPER HEALTH. Tame the party animal inside to once a week and follow your customized program the other 6 days.

4. Keeping that smile

Customer satisfaction requires hard work on your part, listening to their situations, & solving problems. When you have the energy both physically and mentally supporting you, then you will be more alert to respond quicker with action and happier to do so. The more the customer is satisfied, the more $$$ you will earn.

Activity Level   Stress Level
7   7.5

9. LAW ENFORCEMENT & FIREMEN 🚒

It's part of the job!

This professional field goes at two speeds. It is true that there is much downtime spent in this field where your body is at rest. Then, there are moments where sudden bursts of energy are required. Your body has to be ready for "fight or flight" in a moment's notice. This rapid burst of adrenaline allows one to handle some of the worst-case scenarios. Overall, your mental, emotional, and physical strengths need to be at an all-time high when the call of duty arises.

10. *Lifestyle Tips*

Participating in high-intense strength training four days a week with tremendous passion and intensity will be of great benefit and help alleviate the daily stresses. You are a pillar of good character and upholding justice and saving lives in the community so people rely on you for looking strong, acting strong, thinking strong, and eating strong.

Rest is vital for solid mental and physical preparation for the day's activities. Despite the different shifts you may work, you must get that valuable rest in so that you are prepared to go to action. This requires disciplining yourself to get eight hours of sleep a day, everyday.

Bring your all-star foods with you so that you will be alert. This will allow you to take advantage of any downtime by eating nutritiously.

9. *All-Star Foods and Liquid Fuel*

What should you eat at work? What about meals at home? Wherever you are, you must **eat strong!**

Here is a list of top foods to fuel you throughout the day at work and at home:

5 Foods At Work

1. Pure Protein bars, meal replacement powders w/ 1% milk (meal reps replace a regular food meal while adding high-quality nutrients to your body), yogurt (low-fat), Clif bars
2. Grilled chicken breast salads w/ carrots, spinach, tomatoes, cucumbers, leafy greens, olive oil
3. Polly-O stringums lite mozzarella sticks, almonds, sunflower seeds, Brazil nuts
4. Apples, strawberries, peaches, blueberries
5. Fast-food! CAUTION: Our recommendations include:
    a. Subway- chicken breast on wheat bread w/ hot sauce, peppers, lettuce, tomato
    b. Local diner- 8 oz. top round steak, 3 scrambled eggs, 2 slices of whole wheat toast w/ jelly
    c. Wendy's- 2 plain baked potatoes, grilled chicken salad
    d. Boston Market- ¼ white chicken breast, rice pilaf, mixed vegetables

<u>5 Foods At Home</u>
1. **Lean meat**- venison, top round sirloin, flank steak (contain creatine, high in iron & zinc- crucial muscle building nutrients)
2. **Fish**- salmon, herring, cod, mackerel (high in omega 3 fatty acids, contains amino acids necessary for muscle growth, effective in preventing heart disease, improves concentration and mental ability)
3. **Whole-grain cereals** (5/5 rule)- bulgur, barley, fiber one
4. **Sweet potatoes, baked potatoes, mixed veggies, yams, wheat pasta**
5. **Oatmeal & egg whites** (2 yolks)

HOT TIPS:
#1

* Eat 1 gram of protein per pound of what you weigh. Do this consistently to fuel your muscle-building process.

#2

** Drink ½ cup of low-fat milk before bedtime. This helps reduce the amount of protein breakdown that may occur while you sleep.

#3

*** Drink a gallon of water daily.

#4

**** Keep caffeine in moderation.

8. *Foods to Avoid* (🍴 TOP TEN TOPICS, alcohol)
   a. High G.I. carbohydrates (simple sugars)
       white flour products (bagels, pasta, hot dog rolls/hamburger buns, corn bread, English muffins), snacks, cookies, candy, ice cream, soda, granola bars
   b. High trans-fat, saturated fat & hydrogenated oils
       1. fried foods
       2. butter, margarine, cream cheese
           whole milk, cheese
   c. High sodium foods (promote bloating & make you feel sluggish throughout the day)
       1. pizza
       2. Chinese food

        3. frozen entrees
        4. nachos
        5. burritos
    d. Frequent fast food restaurants
        ex. hamburger w/ cheese
        1 medium French fries = 1850 calories
        16 oz. cola soda   (68 g prot/144 g carbs/112 g fat)
    e. Convenience store foods
        1. Chips, burritos, sodas, snacks
        NOTE: The only reason that you will ever stop here and eat is if you don't bring your all-star foods!
    f. On the road pick ups
        1. Grande white chocolate mochas
        2. Grande caffe lattes
        3. Large light and sweet
        4. Donuts, cookies, pastries, bagels
            NOTE: **These are empty, muscle wasting calories.
                **Black coffee w/ some skim milk & sugar substitute in moderation is o.k.

HOT TIP:
#1

*If you need a caffeine kick, there is the same amount of caffeine in a black coffee as the previously stated types of high-calorie drinks above.

7. Meals: How many & when?

Your tank has to be full at all times in case of an emergency situation that will require a great deal of energy expenditure on your part. What does this mean? Your glycogen levels (stored carbohydrates in the muscle) need to be full. Glycogen is the principal storage form of glucose, which is reserved in the muscles and the liver. Digested carbohydrates are processed into simple sugars (glucose), which are then stored as glycogen. When the muscles are satiated with glycogen, they are ready for action.

<u>When should you eat?</u>

Your biggest meal of the day (with the most carbs) should be first thing in the morning or upon waking up (depending on the shift). During your training days, you should have another good-sized meal high in quality carbohydrates within 1-2 hours of training. On your off days from training, cut back on the carbs. Your third meal should be later in the day and should contain a high amount of protein and low carbs. To keep energy up, throughout the day snack on a protein bar or a meal replacement shake if needed.

Breakdown: "the skinny"

MEAL #1- (Most calories) Most carbs, quality protein
Ex. -moderate caffeine, bagel (w/ lite cream cheese), eggs/egg whites, juice

Note: 3 hours later = workout
*Consume meal replacement shake w/banana upon completion of workout

MEAL #2- (2nd largest meal) High in quality carbs & protein
Ex.—Turkey sandwich w/ lettuce and tomato on whole wheat bread

*Consume another meal replacement/protein bar 2-3 hours thereafter

MEAL #3- (smallest meal) Low carbs, high in quality protein
Ex. Grilled chicken salad w/ low-fat dressing & peppers/onions egg white omelet

Lastly, **keep the palate happy & DRINK PLENTY OF WATER!**

6. *Supplementation & Sleep*

What supplements are right for you?

A List

1) multivitamin
2) antioxidant- helps fight free radicals which are a byproduct of intense exercise and a heightened, stressful profession
3) creatine/glutamine- take 5 grams of both first thing in the morning and right after training if your goal is to get stronger and recover from training quicker
4) vitamin B (1000 mg)

B List

1) caffeine- take 200 mg right before training to give you that extra zip
2) NO2
3) ZMA
4) HMB
5) tyrosine, ginseng, ginkgo biloba-these 3 combined aid in mental alertness
6) avoid steroids and prohormones like androstenedione

Firemen

Your sleep may be broken up at times throughout the week. Try to make up for it later in the week by taking short naps or go to bed earlier. The goal is to average around 8 hours of sleep a night. Let your body know that it is sleep deprived and it will repay the favor by hindering your overall fitness goals.

Policemen

Working different shifts often times can lead to inconsistent sleep patterns. Whether you work 1st, 2nd or the midnight shift, get your body conditioned into a regiment of sleeping the same amount at the same time daily. At first this may be challenging, but discipline yourself and after a couple of weeks your body will adapt. You will be able to sleep properly and consequently, function like a well-oiled machine.

5. *Resistance Training* (☕ TOP TEN TOPICS, proper form)

This is essential for this profession because you are faced with many physical challenges. Additionally, this provides a great outlet for reducing stress and looking stronger. By age 25, if we don't resistance train, we begin to lose muscle. Well, if you are climbing the ladder of age and you haven't begun to train yet, no fear! Here is a workout that will challenge these muscles right away and get them back on the track to success.

YOUR WORKOUT:

>   4 day a week
>   3 sets of each exercise
>   MALES: 6-10 reps, going to failure on the final reps of the **last 2 sets**
>   FEMALES: 10-15 reps, going to failure on the final reps of the **last set**

HOT TIP:

#1

*Always warm up your rotator cuffs for 5 minutes before training. Extend your arms straight out to your sides and do 50 small arm circles forward and then follow it up with 50 small arm circles to the rear.

MONDAY: chest & triceps

1) Bench press (flat, barbell)
2) Incline (chest press dumbbells at 20-25 degree bench angle)
3) Straight arm press downs (with cables)
4) Dips (Keep proper form! If need be to challenge yourself, you can add a weighted belt to your own weight.)
5) Standing cable crossovers

TUESDAY: back & biceps

1)   Pull ups (use a weighted belt if your own bodyweight is not challenging enough)
2)   Seated lat rows
3)   Standing barbell curls
4)   Seated dumbbell hammer curls (focus on squeezing an orange between your bicep and your forearm on each rep)
5)   Low back extensions on 45 deg. bench (hold a weight on your chest for a challenge)

WEDNESDAY: day off

THURSDAY: legs

1)   Squats (perform a leg press if you cannot squat with good form. Always have a spotter!)
2)   Step up (use an 18-inch box and hold dumbbells to your side that challenges and forces you to go to failure accordingly)
3)   Lying hamstring curl
4)   Standing calf raises
5)   Leg extensions

FRIDAY: day off

SATURDAY: Shoulders

1)   Seated military press (use dumbbells if you have had shoulder problems)
2)   Seated side lateral raises (raise with your elbows)
3)   Seated reverse pec dec flyes
4)   Stability ball crunches (hold a medicine ball on your chest, for more of a challenge hold directly over your head)
5)   Hanging leg raises (do not use your body weight to gain momentum)

4. *Cardiovascular Training*

INTERVALS, INTERVALS, INTERVALS.

3 days for 20 minutes after resistance training (except on leg day)

DAY 1

Stepmill/Stairmaster

Time	*intensity*	*heart rate*
3 min	easy & slow	65-75%
3 min	hard & fast	75-85%
2 min	easy & slow	65-75%
3 min	hard & fast	80-85%
1 min	easy & slow	65-75%
3 min	hard & fast	80-90%
1 min	easy & slow	65-75%
1 min	hard & fast	85-90%
3 min	easy & slow	60-65%

DAY 2

Windsprints/outdoors

Distance

50 yd dash
70 yd dash
100 yd dash
100 yd dash
100 yd dash   NOTE: After each sprint,
50 yd dash   walk back to the start.
100 yd dash
100 yd dash
50 yd dash
Walk for 1 lap

HOT TIP:
#1

* To incorporate a whole body workout that helps shape your body symmetrically and give that lean look, this is the way to go. This is the fastest way to increase fitness.

#2

*This pattern goes along great with your profession. It forces your body to adapt and recover under stress.

#3

*To help break plateaus in your other training, this will do the trick.

<u>DAY 3</u>

Ergometer (rowing intervals)

<u>*Time*</u>	<u>*Intensity*</u>
3 minute warm up	easy & slow
2 minutes	hard & fast
2 minutes	easy & slow
3 minutes	hard & fast
1 minute	easy & slow
4 minutes	hard & fast
5 minutes	easy & slow

3. Sports

   The sports provided go hand in hand with your training and by training with the program outlined for you, you will be able to excel and perform better in these sports. This is a great outlet for you!

A competitive challenge is always a good thing.

- Flag football league
- Bodybuilding competitions
- Martial arts
- Basketball
- Softball

2. How to Move More   <u>Activity level</u>   <u>7.0</u>

   Your activity level is fairly high because at times you have to work at peak (100%) physical capabilities. There are also instances when your activity level is at a 1 or 2 because of doing paperwork or sitting for prolonged periods of time.

During downtime (especially on slow nights):

    a)   sit with good posture (chest out & spine erect)

                &

    b)   stretch on the hour (bend over & touch toes then extend arms over head as high as possible) **this will take you only 15 seconds**

Many situations are encountered on a daily basis that may put you in awkward positions either sitting, squatting, walking, fighting, running, driving, climbing, etc. Be conscious of your posture to the best of your ability. Draw your navel to your spine and keep your midsection tight.

If you are overweight, perform 1 of the following exercises per hour for every hour of downtime:

    c)   25-30 pushups

    d)   20-25 squats

    e)   50 small arm circles w/ arms out to your side

HOT TIP:
#1

* If you are posed with an extreme, physical situation, after the incident is over and you are in one piece, sit down and reflect on this incident. Write down in a journal what you did well, and how you may have been able to handle the situation differently and rate yourself honestly on a 1-10 scale. Then, the next time that you are faced with a physically and mentally challenging situation, you will be that much more prepared to handle it and give yourself a 10!

1. *Obstacles and Ways To Conquer Them*

1. Eating strong consistently	Day in and day out, stay consistent eating the all-star foods. Bring your meals with you to work, then you won't be faced with a situation where you may have to eat poorly.
2. Training strong consistently	Compete with yourself every time that you go to the gym. Always push your physical limits and you will be amazed at what you can achieve. Attack the weights like a fire or a criminal that you are after in a foot pursuit.

3. High stress level

You have to be physically, mentally, and emotionally like a rock. Use the outlets as discussed (sports/training hard). Leave your job at your job, separate from your home life.

4. Downtime

Take advantage of downtime. Do not become complacent/lazy. Make it time well spent. Focus on your posture. Keep positive thoughts flowing. Mental power is necessary for physical power. Even though it is downtime, you still have to be alert and ready for action.

| | Activity Level | Stress Level |
| | 3.0 | 8.5 |

10. LEGAL 🗁

It's part of the job!

You have paid your dues to get to where you are today! You are more than well versed in the "legaleeze" terminology and how to negotiate with authority on a daily basis. You possess a mental toughness that is exercised many hours throughout the day. Dealing with people and making decisions are things that you do best. Your charisma, wit, intelligence, cunningness, and brashness (when need be), all contribute to you as the showstopper! You are on the phone a lot with important clients and demonstrate a powerful presence.

10. *Lifestyle Tips* (🗁 all TOP TEN TOOLS)

If you are working in a firm, 12-hour days are probably the norm. Encourage your senior partners (or if you are a senior partner) to add a small workout facility into the firm. If the firm you work at is small, then see if you can work out a corporate rate with a nearby gym.

Get yourself in a routine to workout 3 days a week at lunchtime. Schedule your workout as you would for a client. You already have half the battle won with your hard-working, tenacious attitude. Bring this high intense, over-achieving attitude with you to the gym and results will take place in the near future.

If you are working in a courtroom, we advise also to workout during your lunch break. This time to work out is very beneficial for your overall daily performance. You will be re-energized and ready to proceed with a clear focus for each case during the second half of the day.

Separate work from home. If you do work long hours, leave work there. Go home and enjoy the precious time that you have with your family or friends. Then, get to bed and rest up for another day.

You have exercised and will continue to exercise your mind to great lengths. Don't forget to condition the physical side of your body as well. Much of your day may be attributed to sitting and analyzing information for work meetings. Getting in a consistent weekly training regiment will bring you one step closer to SUPER HEALTH! Looking fit & healthy will help your powerful image and as a judge or prosecution/defense attorneys, this can make a big difference.

Bring your all-star foods with you to work and have control over when & where you eat. Rather than going for a power lunch to a fine dining establishment eating rich, fatty foods, appetizers, alcoholic beverages, desserts, etc., keep your eye on the prize that you brought with you. Remember to drink your recommended amounts of water.

9. All-Star Foods and Liquid Fuel

<u>FOODS AT WORK</u>

Pure Protein bars	**Clif bars**
Luna bars	**Fiberone cereal**
Grapenuts cereal	**sunflower seeds**
peanuts	**Brazil nuts**
pumpkin seeds	**12 oz. water**

➢ Good salad choices:
- o Cobb salad
- o Three-bean salads
- o Fruit salad
- o Tomato salad
- o Tossed salad w/ shrimp, olives, cucumbers, olive oil & vinegar

➢ pepper turkey breast (6 oz.) on pumpernickel, deli pickle

<u>ALL-STAR SNACKS</u>

➢ Dried fruits, raisins, low-fat yogurt, cottage cheese, hard-boiled eggs, oranges

<u>FOODS AT HOME</u>

➢ Old-fashioned oatmeal, 4 egg whites, 1 yolk, orange juice, grapefruit
➢ Grilled chicken breast, 1 cup-brown rice, 2 cups-mixed veggies
➢ Top round sirloin (grilled), sweet potato (baked), carrot sticks
➢ Albacore canned tuna fish on rye bread, 1 cup-cooked spinach
➢ Veggie burger, pearl barley, mushroom kabobs
➢ Salmon (6-8 oz.), tomato-flavored couscous, asparagus
➢ Swordfish, brown rice, baked beans

<u>FOODS AT THE RESTAURANT</u>

Tips for restaurant dining:

1) No alcohol consumption. Replace w/ 12 oz. water.
2) No appetizers or desserts

3) Order grilled, baked, or broiled foods
4) Avoid creamy dressings or cheese at the salad bar
5) Order vegetables instead of carbs for sides
6) Sushi is a high protein, mentality enhancer

Liquid Fuel

- WATER! (of course)- 12 oz. w/ meal
- Decaffeinated herbal tea
- Decaffeinated coffee

8. *Foods to Avoid*

Foods high in sugar

chocolate	muffins
soda	donuts
cookies	pasta
hoagie rolls	white rice
macaroni & cheese	pancakes w/ strawberry topping
chips	cereals (over 5 grams of sugar)

Foods high in trans fat

On the back of nutritional labels, they are now indicating the amount of trans fat in a specific product. Check this label and avoid foods high in trans fat.

nachos	high-calorie, high-fat creamy salad
croutons	dressings
pre-made dips	frozen entrees
processed dinner aids	foods w/ "hydrogenated" vegetable oil
whipped dessert toppings	as an ingredient

Late night binge foods

pasta	cheeseburgers & bacon
pizza & beer	sloppy joes
meatball grinders on white bread	
chicken parmigiana	

Restaurant forbiddens

appetizers	desserts
alcohol	coffee w/ cream & sugar
fried foods	bagels, hotcakes, biscuits, homefries
luncheon meats (pastrami, salami, bologna) at local delis	
big bowls of pasta	

7. *Meals: How many & when?*

Relax and read the daily newspaper and see who made the infamous list in the police blotter (as an attorney, these may be people that you will be representing) or see if your favorite baseball team won while eating your breakfast. Make certain that you get the day started correctly by eating a sound breakfast. Keep the fuel tank around full throughout the day by eating small servings every 3 hours.

Keep your all-star foods close by (in the car, office, on your person with you). Consume a moderate lunch within 1 hour of your workout. DO NOT eat past 8 P.M. You may get so entrenched in your work that day that you lose track of time and end up going all day barely eating anything. This will set you up for inevitable physical and mental failure.

So here is the breakdown:

1. A good sound, nutritious breakfast
2. A small meal or snack around 10:30 am
3. A moderate lunch within 1 hour of your workout
4. A small meal or snack around 3 pm
5. A good sound, nutritious dinner no later that 8 pm

6. *Supplementation & Sleep*

With your high stress level (8.5), you must go to bed the same time each night for an average of 7 hours during the workweek and 8-9 hours a night on your days off. Without proper rest, you aren't much benefit to your clients, family, friends or yourself for that matter. Take care of yourself first and then you will have a more relaxed state of mind with the ability to formulate and communicate clear, wise decisions. You will have a better patience for handling difficult tasks and your aura as a leader will really start to beam brightly!

What supplements are right for you?
A List

1. multivitamin
2. antioxidant

3. melatonin
4. vitamin B (100 mg)
5. meal replacement

<u>**B** List</u>

1. glutamine
2. caffeine (only 150 mg. before training)

5. Resistance Training
   A strong, lean physique will present a great image. Overcoming physical challenges in the gym will help you conquer any mental challenges that come your way in cases, negotiations, or other problems.

A workout right for you!

- Monday/Wednesday/Friday
- Lunchtime is the ideal time

<u>MONDAY</u> (upper body)

- ❑ Superset workout
- ❑ 3 total sets/exercise
- ❑ 2 exercises back to back with no rest in between
- ❑ One minute rest between supersets
- ❑ FEMALES: 12-15 reps, 80-90% failure on last 2 reps
  MALES: 10-12 reps, 80-99% failure on last 2 reps

*Warm up with 50 arm circles to the front & 50 arm circles to the rear.

1) Machine chest press
2) Seated lat row
   1 MIN REST
3) Machine chest press
4) Seated lat row
   1 MIN REST
5) Machine chest press
6) Seated lat row
   1 MIN REST

- Perform the same scheme for the following paired exercises

    1) Standing barbell curl
    2) Lying dumbbell tricep extensions

    1) Incline dumbbell press
    2) Side lateral raises

    1) Seated dumbbell shoulder press
    2) Lat pulldowns

    1) Low back extensions
    2) Hanging leg raises

HOT TIP:
#1

*This workout is good for the novice all the way to the experienced. Start with a weight that you will go to failure with in the correct number of repetitions. With time, challenge yourself and you will notice yourself climbing the SUPER HEALTH ladder from novice to seasoned to advanced to elite to the peak of wellness!

#2

*Put a gym into your law firm and get everyone there into the healthful spirit. You will no longer have to leave the office to workout. On the other hand, savvy lawyers may want to set up a corporate account w/ a local gym and workout with some other business partners.

<u>WEDNESDAY (lower body)</u>

NOTE: Follow the same repetition scheme and supersetting sequence as for the upper body workout.

*Warm up with 15 body weight squats

    1) Lying leg press
    2) Stationary lunges (alternate legs)

    1) Lying leg curls
    2) Seated leg curls

1) Seated leg extensions
2) Step ups on 18 inch box (alternate legs)

1) Seated calf raises
2) Standing calf raises

1) Stability ball crunches
2) Wall squat (1 minute)

FRIDAY (total body)

NOTE: Follow the same repetition scheme and supersetting sequence as for the upper & lower body workouts. In addition, you will incorporate an aerobic third component of the superset making this a triset. For this workout, there will be no rest between exercises, but a 1 minute rest between trisets.

*Warm up with 15 body weight squats, 25 arm circles to the front & rear.

1) Dumbbell chest press
2) Lying leg press
3) Jump rope-1 minute

1) Seated lat row
2) Lying leg curl
3) Stepmill-2 minutes

1) Seated dumbbell bicep curls
2) Leg extensions
3) Jumping jacks-1 minute

1) Seated machine shoulder press
2) Wall squat
3) Treadmill run (7.5 mph)-3 minutes

1) Hanging leg raises
2) Stability ball crunches
3) X-trainer elliptical-4 minutes

4. Cardiovascular training

- ❑ **2 days a week (Mon/Wed) for 15 minutes**
- ❑ **Perform intervals following resistance training**

<u>MONDAY</u> (x-trainer elliptical)

TIME	INTERVAL	HEART RATE
3 min	low & slow	60-65%
2 min	fast & hard	80-85%

REPEAT THIS 3 TIMES (for 15 minutes)

<u>WEDNESDAY</u> (stepmill)

TIME	INTERVAL	HEART RATE
3 min	low & slow	60-65%
2 min	fast & hard	80-85%

REPEAT THIS 3 TIMES (for 15 minutes)

Are you aspiring for more healthy heart-pounding fun?

**Perform one extra lunchtime cardio workout for 45 minutes. Go outside and take a brisk walk (HR 60-65%). This will be great for clearing the cobwebs from your mind!

3. Sports

   We recommend Tuesday & Thursday during lunchtime to get the competitive juices flowing. This will get you into a great weekly routine for ultimate SUPER HEALTH. If during the week is just not feasible, get out during the weekend early in the morning and join some friends for some "friendly competition".

Great competitive sports for you!

- Pick up basketball games at the local YMCA
- Racquetball
- Golf (walk or have a caddy carry your clubs for some friendly "skins" competition)
- Yoga, Pilates, Tai Chi

2. How to Move More   <u>Activity level</u>   <u>3.0</u>

If you are sitting by your desk all day, simply get up and away from the "world of inactivity". Here are some things you can do to help you better move while in the office.

- Get social and visit your co-workers
- Go to the restroom
- Do 15 body weight squats
- Touch sky, touch toe stretch
- Do 15 pushups

Your intensity can be high at times and your stress levels can build.

Don't lose your temper. Play it cool by taking a walk away from the stressful environment. Get off of the phone & sit in peace. Post positive sayings in your office and have some ultimate relaxations, like music, playing. Keep handgrips in your office to squeeze out all of the built up tension. If you are a golf nut, have a putter handy to putt some golf balls into a cup. Whatever you do, don't let the stress mount up day after day. Find what works best for you and stick to it!

1. Obstacles and Ways To Conquer Them

1. Finding time for working out	Plan your lunchtime workouts into your weekly schedule. You will come to look forward to this appointment as the best part of the day. You will do very well for your health. Keep the intensity and passion high. Again, if conducive, invest in implementing a gym into the office.
2. Eating out (w/ clients)	Stick strongly to our top tips that we set specifically for you. Stay disciplined and feed your body what it deserves from the all-star food selection list. You are a natural born leader; so then, lead the way to a more physically & nutritionally conscious YOU!
3. Separating work from home	If you do work 12-16 hours a day regularly, your mind could easily live at work. Don't let that happen! You need a balance & harmony in your life for overall wellness. You are an integral person in many lives, so be a role model and get the proper rest and fuel necessary. Encourage loved ones to join the SUPER HEALTH club! Your influence runs deep to make a difference!

4. Exercising

You have to realize that your well being is the most important thing to you, personally. Without health, what do you have? You certainly realize that it took hard work and determination mentally to make it as a superior professional in what you do & that you had to conquer many obstacles set forth in your path. The same principle pertains to the exercise & fitness arena. You can go & achieve at lengths what you choose based on your work ethic in training, eating, & resting. You can and will do it. We rest our case! This court is adjourned!

CHEST

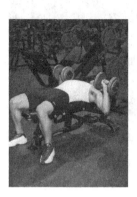 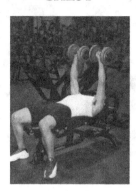

1. Dumbbell Bench Press (Flat Bench)

1. Lie on your back on a flat bench holding a dumbbell in each hand.
2. Palms are facing your feet.
3. Elbows are out to your side.
4. Stay strong on your heels.
5. Keep your hips & buttocks firmly on the bench.
6. Push the dumbbells straight up and together across the middle of your chest not letting the dumbbells touch.
7. 1 second on the way up, exhaling.
8. Pause for 1 second at the top, squeezing your chest muscles.
9. Control the dumbbells and lower them back to the starting position.
10. 2 seconds on the way down, inhaling.

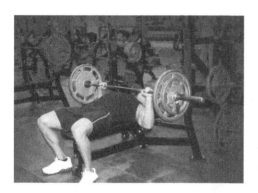 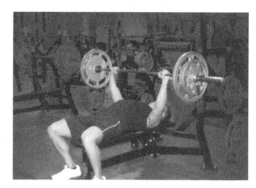

2. Flat Barbell Bench Press

1. Lie on your back on a flat bench and firmly position your feet flat on the ground.
2. Keep your hips and buttocks firmly on the bench. Arch your back slightly and raise your chest high.
3. Grab the bar with a slightly wider than shoulder width grip.
4. Bring the barbell down to the middle portion of your chest, just above chest level (1/2 inch).
5. Keep your elbows out to the side.
6. Inhale for 2 seconds on the way down.
7. Get "under" the barbell.
8. Press up strongly with your chest.
9. Straighten your arms at the top without locking out your elbows.
10. Exhale for 1 second on the way up.

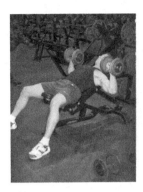 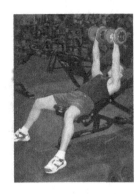

3. Dumbbell Incline Press

1. Adjust the bench so that it is at a 15-20 degree angle.
2. Pick up dumbbells with each hand and place them on your thighs.
3. Position them at the base of your shoulders.
4. Press the dumbbells up and over your chest.
5. Bring the dumbbells together at the top of the exercise without letting the dumbbells hit.
6. Squeeze your chest at the top of the movement pausing for 1 second.
7. Exhale for 1 second on the way up.
8. Control the dumbbells and slowly lower to start position.
9. Keep tension in the chest muscles while lowering the weight.
10. Inhale for 2 seconds on the way down.

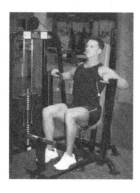 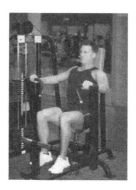

4. Machine Chest Press

1. Sit on the chair with your feet firmly placed on the ground.
2. Sit up tall keeping your chest up, shoulders back, and abs tight.
3. Grab the handles broader than shoulder width.
4. Your elbows and wrists should be lined up with each other.
5. Push forcefully with your chest muscles.
6. Exhale for 1 second on the push.
7. Pause for 1 second at the end of the press squeezing your chest muscles.
8. Control the weight and bring back to the start position.
9. Keep tension in the chest muscles while lowering the weight.
10. Inhale for 2 seconds on the way down.

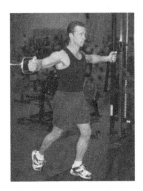 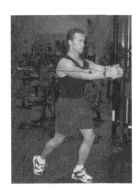

5.   Standing Cable Crossovers

1.   Align the handles and cable line with the middle of your chest.
2.   Place one foot in front of the other with slightly bent knees.
3.   Grab the handles as your would a dumbbell.
4.   Stand up tall.
5.   Start the exercise just as you would with dumbbells with your elbows in line with wrists.
6.   Push the handles straight in front of you across your chest.
7.   Exhale for 1 second on the push.
8.   Pause for 1 second, squeeze the chest muscles at the end of the press.
9.   Control the cables and handles and return to starting position.
10. Exhale for 2 seconds on the way down.

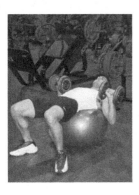 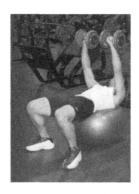

6. Dumbbell Bench Press (on stability ball)

1. Pretend the ball is a bench.
2. Keep your feet directly below your knees with your thighs parallel to the floor.
3. Keep your shoulder blades on the stability ball.
4. Keep your abs tight.
5. Push the dumbbells straight up and together across the middle of your chest not letting the dumbbells touch.
6. Exhale for 1 second on the way down.
7. Pause for 1 second at the top, squeezing your chest and controlling your body and dumbbells.
8. Lower dumbbells back to the starting position.
9. Inhale for 2 seconds on the way down.
10. Keep constant tension in your chest on the way down and keep your strong base.

BACK

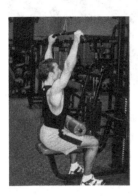 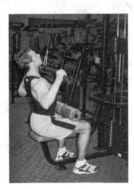

1. Seated Lat Pulldowns

1. Secure your legs in the seat, staying strong on your heels.
2. Grab the bar overhead with a slightly wider than shoulder width grip.
3. Arch your back slightly from the waist, keeping your chest up.
4. Pull the bar down just below chin level with your back muscles.
5. Think of your arms as hooks and try not to pull with them.
6. Exhale for 1 second on the way down.
7. Pause for 1 second at the bottom squeezing your back muscles.
8. Control the weight on the way up, keeping the tension in the back muscles.
9. Keep your upper body tight in the same position you started the exercise.
10. Inhale for 2 seconds on the way up.

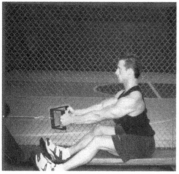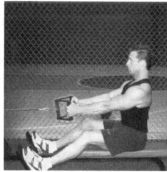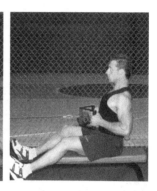

2. Seated Lat Rows

1. Sit with your feet placed firmly on the foot rests, strong on your heels with a slight bend in the knees.
2. Grab a bar handle that is shoulder width apart.
3. Sit up tall with your chest up high, shoulders back, and slightly arched back from the waist.
4. Pull the bar to your bellybutton squeezing your shoulder blades together.
5. Pull with your elbows using your back muscles.
6. Exhale for 1 second on the pull.
7. Pause for 1 second at full contraction squeezing your back muscles.
8. Control the weight with your back muscles, maintaining good posture. Return to start.
9. Do not let the weight move your upper body. You control the weight.
10. Inhale for 2 seconds on the way down.

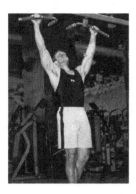 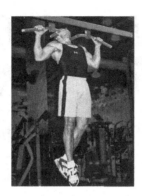

3. Pullups.

1. Grab the pullup bar with a slightly wider than shoulder width grip.
2. Maintain good posture while keeping your arms straight.
3. Keep a slight bend in the knees.
4. Arch your back slightly from the waist.
5. Pull yourself up so that your chin is above the bar. Pause for 1 second squeezing your back muscles.
6. Exhale for 1 second on the way up.
7. Control your body. Do not bounce, swing, or use momentum.
8. Lower your body, keeping tension in the back muscles.
9. Bring your body to the starting position.
10. Inhale for two seconds on the way down.

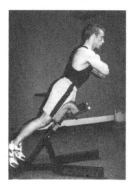 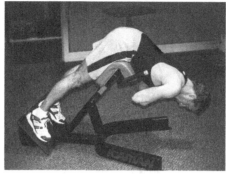

4. Low Back Extensions

1. Lean against the pad at the waist so free movement of your upper body is allowed.
2. Secure ankles against the back foot padding for support with feet flat on surface.
3. Keep your body straight with good posture as if you were standing up.
4. Place arms across chest (or out in front-advanced).
5. Roll shoulders forward and extend upper body down from the waist.
6. Focus on the low back stretching and extending (don't go too low).
7. Inhale for 2 seconds on the way down.
8. Contract low back muscles and raise upper body to start position.
9. Control body, focus on keeping constant tension in the low back. Do not bounce.
10. Exhale for 2 seconds on the way up and pause for 1 second at the top squeezing your lower back muscles.

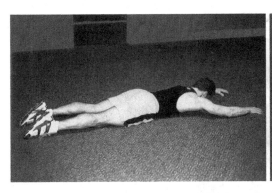 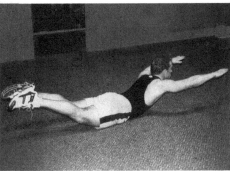

5. Supermans

1. Lie flat on stomach with arms in front of you.
2. Using low back muscles raise legs, feet, arms, and hands approximately 4-6 inches off of the ground.
3. Exhale for 1 second on the way up.
4. Pause for 3 seconds at the top flexing your low back muscles.
5. Inhale for 1 second while lowering your body to starting position. Repeat.

BICEPS

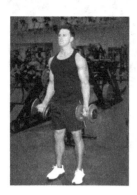 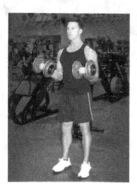

1. Dumbbell Bicep Curls

1. Stand with feet shoulder width apart.
2. Grab a pair of dumbbells. Palms up toward the sky, thumbs out and arms fully extended.
3. Slightly bend knees. Keep head and chest up, shoulders back, and abs tight.
4. Curl the dumbbells to full contraction to the middle of chest.
5. Squeeze your biceps fully.
6. Exhale for 1 second on the way up.
7. Pause for 1 second at full contraction.
8. Control the weight with biceps. Do not rock your body to gather momentum.
9. Maintain tension on biceps as you lower the weight.
10. Inhale for 2 seconds on the way down.

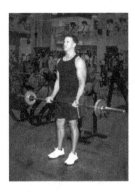 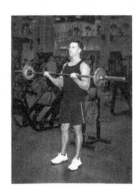

2. Barbell Bicep Curls

1. Stand with feet shoulder width apart.
2. Grab the barbell with palms up, arms straight down where they fall naturally from the shoulders.
3. Slightly bend knees, keeping head up, chest out, shoulders back, and abs tight.
4. Curl the barbell to full contraction of the bicep to the middle of the chest.
5. Squeeze biceps fully.
6. Exhale for 1 second on the way up.
7. Pause for 1 second at full contraction.
8. Control the weight with biceps. Do not rock your body to gather momentum.
9. Maintain tension on biceps as you lower the weight.
10. Inhale for 2 seconds on the way down.

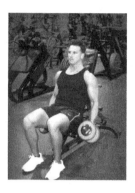 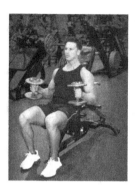

3. Incline Seated Hammer Curls

1. Adjust the incline bench to approximately 75-80 degrees.
2. Grab a pair of dumbbells with palms each other and thumbs at the top.
3. Keep head up, shoulders back, arms straight down, and stay strong on your heels.
4. Curl the dumbbells to full contraction to the middle of chest.
5. Squeeze biceps and forearms fully.
6. Exhale for 1 second on the way up.
7. Pause for 1 second at full contraction.
8. Control the weights with arm muscles.
9. Maintain tension on biceps and forearms on the way down.
10. Inhale for 2 seconds on the way down.

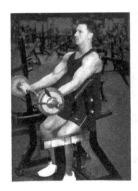 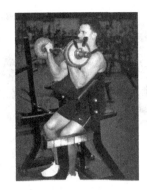

4. Preacher Curls

1. Adjust the seat so that your feet are flat on the ground/machine.
2. Grab the cambered barbell keeping elbows firm against the pad.
3. Keep head up, shoulders back while holding the bar at the top in a flexed position.
4. Lower the barbell slowly, keeping all tension on biceps.
5. Keep elbows on the pad and maintain a tension in the low back muscles.
6. Inhale for 2 seconds on the way down.
7. Contract biceps and raise to the start position.
8. Control the weight and lift with biceps.
9. Pretend as if you were flexing your biceps in the mirror.
10. Exhale for 1 second on the way up.

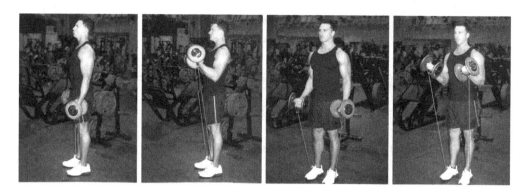

5. Dumbbell Curls (with tubing)

1. Stand with feet shoulder width apart. Wrap tubing under your feet.
2. Hold the tubing handles in each hand with a dumbbell in each hand, also.
3. Slightly bend your knees, keep chest up, shoulders back, arms straight.
4. Curl the dumbbells/tubing handles to full contraction to the middle-to-upper portion of your chest.
5. Squeeze biceps completely.
6. Exhale for 2 seconds on the way up.
7. Pause for 1 second at full contraction.
8. Control the dumbbells/tubing on the way down. Do not rock your body.
9. Maintain tension on biceps as you lower the weight.
10. Inhale for 2 seconds on the way down.

TRICEPS

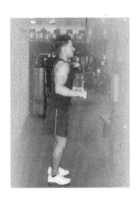 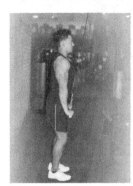

1. Standing Tricep Pressdowns

1. Stand in front of the cables with feet shoulder width apart.
2. Use a cambered bar and place hands shoulder width apart.
3. Slightly bend knees. Keep chest up and begin with elbows bent.
4. Press down and straighten your arms extending the elbows.
5. Focus on using your triceps and flex them at the bottom.
6. Exhale for 1 second on the way down.
7. Pause for 1 second at full contraction.
8. Control the weight with your triceps, keeping body stable. Abs and legs stay strong.
9. Maintain tension on triceps as you raise the bar to the starting position.
10. Inhale for 2 seconds on the way up.

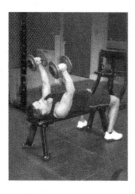 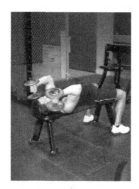

2. Lying Dumbbell Extensions

1. Lie on your back on a flat bench holding a dumbbell in each hand with your arms straight up over you.
2. Palms are facing each other.
3. Stay strong on your heels.
4. Keep shoulders, hips, and buttocks firmly on the bench.
5. Lower the dumbbells in a controlled fashion straight down from the starting position.
6. Maintain tension on triceps while lowering the weight just past your head.
7. Inhale for 3 seconds on the way down.
8. Continue to keep your firm base on the bench. Keep elbows steady. The only body parts moving are your arms.
9. Extend arms straight up to the starting position using your triceps.
10. Exhale for 1 second on the way up.

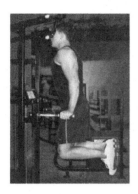 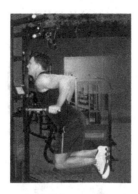

3. Dips

1. Use a dip bar that is shoulder width apart.
2. Hop up on it and begin with your arms straight and knees bent.
3. Keep chest up, abs, tight, head and shoulders back.
4. Start to lower your body by bending your elbows and keeping your body straight up and down.
5. Keep chest up, use triceps to lower your body so your arms finish parallel to the ground.
6. Inhale for 3 seconds on the way down.
7. Push your body back up to the starting position using your triceps.
8. Keep your body straight up and down (without leaning forward or backwards)
9. Exhale for 1 second on the way up.
10. Pause for 1 second at the top.

SHOULDERS

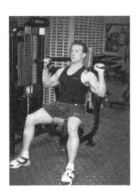 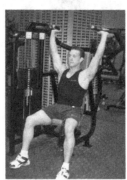

1. Machine Shoulder Press

1. Sit on the chair with your feet firmly on the ground.
2. Sit up tall, keeping head back, chest up, abs tight, and strong on your heels.
3. Push up with your shoulder muscles.
4. Exhale for 1 second on the way up.
5. Extend your arms up without straightening them. Never lock out the elbows.
6. Lower the weight slowly controlling the weight with your shoulder muscles.
7. Maintain constant tension on shoulders on the way down.
8. Inhale for 2 seconds on the way down.
9. Pause for 1 second.
10. Repeat. Always control the weight.

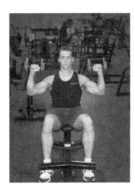 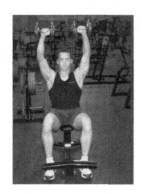

2. Seated Dumbbell Shoulder Press

1. Adjust the bench so that the bench is approximately 75-80 degrees.
2. Place each dumbbell on each of your thighs.
3. Bring the dumbbells overhead. Never lock out the elbows.
4. Lower the dumbbells slowly with your elbows out to your side. Keep tension on shoulders.
5. Lower your elbows just below chest level.
6. Inhale for 2 seconds on the way down.
7. Pause for 1 second at the bottom, tensing your shoulders.
8. Press the dumbbells straight up using your shoulders.
9. Press the dumbbells straight up just before you straighten your arms.
10. Exhale for 1 second on the way up.

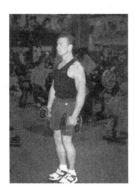 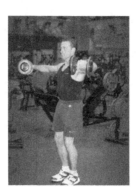

3. Side Raises with Dumbbells

1. Stand with your feet shoulder width apart with a slight bend in the knees.
2. Hold a pair of dumbbells at your side with palms facing each other.
3. Keep your chest up, abs tight, head up, and low back and legs strong.
4. Raise the dumbbells out the side of your body.
5. Raise the dumbbells with your elbows using your shoulder muscles up to parallel to the floor.
6. Exhale for 2 seconds on the way up.
7. Pause for 1 second at the top, tensing your shoulders.
8. Control the dumbbells and lower slowly keeping tension on shoulders.
9. Bring the dumbbells back to the starting position without using momentum.
10. Inhale for 2 seconds on the way down.

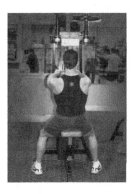 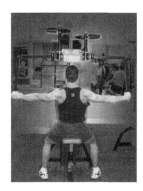

4. Seated Reverse Flyes

1. Sit with your chest up against the backrest and feet flat on the floor.
2. Line up the handles with your shoulders. Arms should be parallel to the floor.
3. Keep your chest up, head neutral, low back and legs strong.
4. Using your elbows and keeping your arms straight pull the handles out to the side and towards the rear of your body.
5. Keep the rear part of your shoulders tense and pull the weight with this part.
6. Exhale for 2 seconds on the pull.
7. Pause for 1 second at full contraction, where your arms should be straight out to the side.
8. Control the weight with your rear shoulder muscles, keeping the tension in this area.
9. Lower the weight and bring the handles back to the starting position using your elbows.
10. Inhale for 2 seconds on the way back to the starting position.

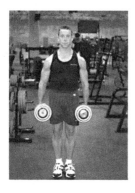 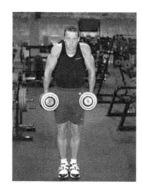

5. Dumbbell Shrugs

1. Stand with feet shoulder width apart with a slight bend in the knees.
2. Grab a pair of dumbbells and drop your hands straight down to your sides. Shift weights slightly in front of your body.
3. Keep head up, chest up, abs tight and begin to tense trapezius muscles.
4. Raise the dumbbells up while keeping arms straight (slight bend in elbows).
5. Pull with your trap muscles, visualize as if you were pulling your shoulders up to your ears.
6. Exhale for 1 second on the way up.
7. Pause for 1 second at the top, squeezing trap muscles.
8. Control the dumbbells with traps and refrain from any rocking motion.
9. Lower the weights to the starting position keeping all of the tension on traps.
10. Inhale for 2 seconds on the way down.

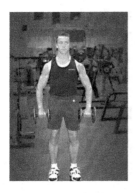 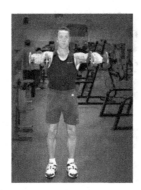

6. Front Raises

1. Stand with your feet shoulder width apart with a slight bend in the knees.
2. Grab a pair of dumbbells and hold them in front of you with palms facing each other.
3. Keep chest up, abs tight, head up, low back and legs strong.
4. Raise the dumbbells up in front of your body using your elbows.
5. Raise the dumbbells up so that your arms are parallel to the floor in front of you.
6. Exhale for 2 seconds on the way up flexing your shoulder muscles.
7. Pause for 1 second at the top flexing your shoulder muscles.
8. Control the dumbbells with your shoulders and keep your body motionless.
9. Lower the dumbbells down to your starting position keeping tension on the shoulders.
10. Inhale for 2 seconds on the way down.

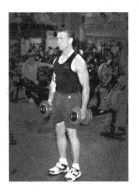 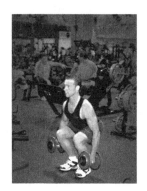 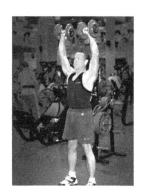

7. Squat Thrusts

1. Stand with your feet shoulder width apart with good posture.
2. Grab a pair of dumbbells and hold them down to your side.
3. Squat down so that your thighs are parallel to the floor, arms remaining out to your side with dumbbells in hand.
4. Inhale for 2 seconds on the way down tensing your leg muscles.
5. Explode up using your legs while simultaneously pressing the dumbbells overhead.
6. Use your legs to begin the thrust and then shoulders to press the dumbbells overhead.
7. Keep your body controlled and do not use momentum.
8. Exhale for 1 second on the way up.
9. Pause for 1 second at the top while tensing your shoulders and maintaining good posture.
10. Bring the dumbbells back down to the start position with your arms down at your sides.

LEGS

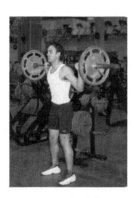 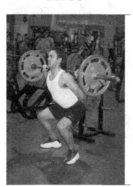

1. Barbell Squats

1. Stand with your feet flat and slightly wider than shoulder width apart with the bar placed evenly on the back of your shoulders.
2. Stand with good posture. Begin to tense your legs and keep abs tight.
3. Squat down extending your hips back, while keeping your chest and head up.
4. Pretend as if you are sitting in a chair, keeping your legs tense.
5. Squat down until your thighs are about parallel to the floor, keeping your head up, chest up, and abs tight.
6. Inhale for 3 seconds on the way down.
7. Do not bounce at the bottom, keeping all of the tension in your leg muscles.
8. Extend knees and hips up until legs are straight using your leg muscles.
9. Exhale for 1 second on the way up, flexing and tensing legs.
10. Pause for 1 second at the top, maintaining good posture.

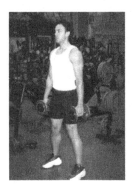 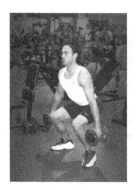

2. Dumbbell Squats

1. Stand with your feet slightly wider than shoulder width apart, standing with good posture.
2. Stand with the dumbbells grasped to your sides.
3. Squat down extending your hips back while keeping your chest and head up.
4. Descend until your thighs are parallel to the floor.
5. Keep chest up, head up, abs tight, and keep all the tension on the thighs.
6. Inhale for 3 seconds on the way down.
7. Do not bounce at the bottom, keeping all the tension on your leg muscles.
8. Extend your knees and hips up until your legs are straight using your leg muscles.
9. Exhale for 1 second on the way up, tensing your leg muscles.
10. Pause for 1 second at the top, maintaining good posture.

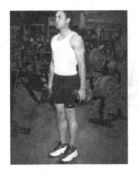 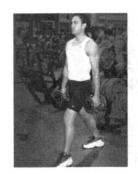 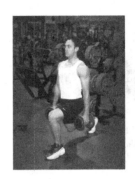

3. Stationary Lunges

1. Stand with dumbbells grasped to your sides. Feet should be shoulder width apart.
2. Keep torso upright throughout the exercise.
3. Lunge forward with your first leg, landing on your heal and then forefoot.
4. Lower your body by flexing your knee and hip of your front leg until the knee of your rear leg is almost hitting the floor. Front leg's knee should not go in front of the plane of your front leg's toes (to prevent knee strain).
5. Inhale for 2 seconds on the way down.
6. Return to the original starting position by forcibly extending your hip and knee of your front (lunge) leg.
7. Exhale for 1 second on the way up.
8. Pause for 1 second at the top, eliminating any momentum.
9. Perform the same sequence for the opposing leg.
10. This counts as 1 repetition combined after working both legs once.

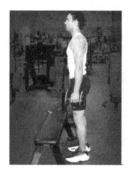 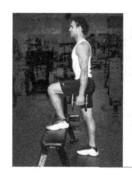 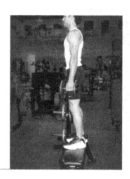

4. Stepups

1. Set up a step (or a sound box) that is 16-18 inches off of the ground.
2. Position yourself in front of the step with the weights grasped to your sides, feet shoulder width apart.
3. Keep your torso upright throughout the exercise.
4. Step up with your left foot and flex your knee and hip of this left leg and forcefully step up with this leg bringing your right foot on the step.
5. Exhale for 1 second on the way up.
6. Step down with your left foot first, then step down with your right foot.
7. Inhale for 1 second on the way down.
8. Pause for 1 second at the bottom, eliminating any momentum.
9. Perform the given number of repetitions for this same leg.
10. After performing the repetitions with the left leg, do the same for the right leg.

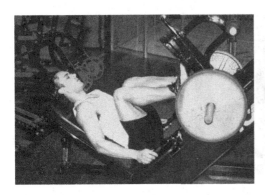 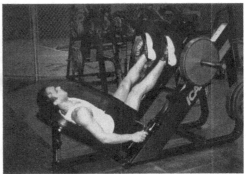

5. Leg Press

1. Sit on machine with back on padded support. Keep torso upright.
2. Place feet on platform shoulder width apart. Grasp handles on the side.
3. Start with your hips and knees extended straight up, but do not lock your knees.
4. Lower the sled by flexing your hips and knees until your knees are just shy of complete flexion, keeping tension in your thighs.
5. Inhale for 2 seconds on the way down.
6. Extend your knees and hips back to the starting position using your thighs.
7. Push with your heels.
8. Exhale for 2 seconds on the way up.
9. Do not lock your knees at the top.
10. Pause for 1 second at the top, keeping tension on your thighs.

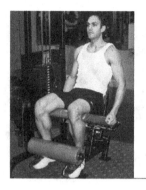 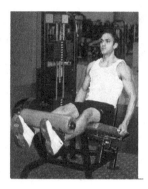

6. Leg Extensions

1. Sit on the machine with your back against the padded support.
2. Sit with your torso erect, grasping the handles to your sides.
3. Place the front of your lower legs under the padded lever.
4. Position your knee joint in line with the same axis as the lever fulcrum.
5. Move the lower level forward by extending your knees until your legs are straight.
6. Legs should be parallel to the floor at the top.
7. Exhale for 1 second on the way up using your lower thighs.
8. Pause for 1 second at the top, squeezing your lower thighs.
9. Return the lower level to the original position by bending your knees.
10. Inhale for 2 seconds on the way down, keeping tension on your legs.

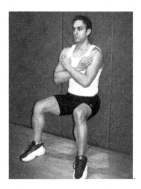

7. Wall Squats

1. Position your body against the wall with you seated, thighs are parallel to the floor.
2. Keep your torso up and legs slightly wider than shoulder width apart.
3. Keep all of the tension in your legs.
4. Hold against the wall as long as possible.

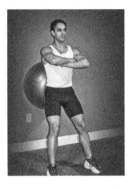 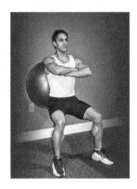

8. Wall Squats (with ball)

1.   Place the stability ball against the wall.
2.   Stand in front with your low back firmly against the ball.
3.   Feet shoulder width apart, keeping your torso erect.
4.   Squat down extending your hips back, keeping tension on the thighs.
5.   Squat down until thighs are parallel to the floor, sliding your torso over the ball.
6.   Inhale for 2 seconds on the way down.
7.   Pause for 1 second at the bottom, keeping tension on the thighs.
8.   Push your body straight up with leg muscles.
9.   Keep torso erect and against the ball.
10. Exhale for 1 second on the way up.

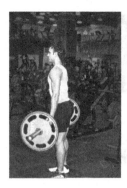 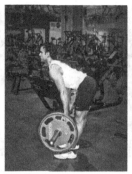 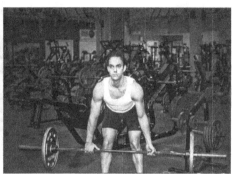

9. Straight Leg Deadlifts

1. Stand with your feet shoulder width apart with your torso erect.
2. Hold the barbell in front of you with your hands on the barbell. One hand is in the pronated (palms downward) position while the other hand is in the supinated (palms upward) position.
3. With your knees straight, lower the bar by bending your hips or pushing them back until your hamstrings feel stretched.
4. Do not bend your lower back, keep chest up, shoulders back and head up at the bottom of the movement.
5. Inhale for 3 seconds on the way down.
6. Keep all the tension in the hamstrings throughout the exercise.
7. Lift the bar by extending your hips until your body is upright.
8. Pull your shoulders slightly back at the top of the lift.
9. Exhale for 1 second on the up.
10. Pause for 1 second at the top squeezing your hamstrings and keeping your torso upright. Tension should not be felt in the lower back throughout this exercise.

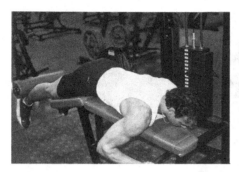 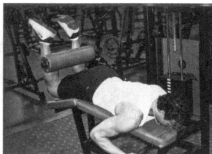

10. Lying Leg Curls

1. Lie prone on the bench with your knees just past the edge of the bench.
2. Put your lower legs under the lever pads and grasp the handles, keeping your head up.
3. Begin to tense your hamstrings.
4. Raise the lever pads to the top of your hamstrings and buttocks.
5. Exhale for 2 seconds while squeezing your hamstrings on the way up.
6. Pause for 1 second at the top, keeping tension on the hamstrings.
7. Lower the lever pads until your knees are straight.
8. Maintain constant tension on the hamstrings while lowering the lever.
9. Do not rock or move your upper body at all.
10. Inhale for 2 seconds on the way down.

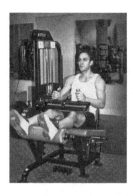 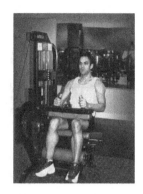

11. Seated Leg Curls

1. Sit on the apparatus with your back against the back support, keeping your torso in an upright position.
2. Place the back of your lower legs (lower calves) on top of the padded lever.
3. Secure the lap pad against your thighs just above your knees giving you your starting position, along with grasping the handles on your lap support.
4. Pull the lever down towards your hamstrings by using your hamstrings and flexing your knees.
5. Exhale for 2 seconds on the way down.
6. Pause for 1 second at the bottom, squeezing your hamstrings.
7. Maintain constant tension on the hamstrings.
8. Return the lever until your legs are straight at the top.
9. Keep tension on hamstrings on the way up.
10. Inhale for 2 seconds on the way up.

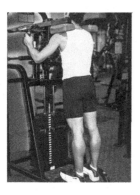 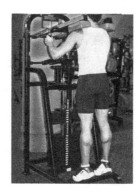

12. Standing Calf Raises

1. Stand with your shoulders squarely under the pads and the balls of your feet are on the platform shoulder width apart.
2. Keep your torso erect and head up. Lock hips and knees.
3. Keep toes pointed forward and begin to tense your calf raises.
4. Raise your heels and stand as tall as possible. Focus on your calves doing all of the work when raising up on the balls of your feet.
5. Exhale for 2 seconds on the way up.
6. Pause for 2 seconds at the top, squeezing and keeping the contraction in your calf muscles.
7. Lower your heels as far as possible, below the platform until you feel a good stretch in the calf muscles.
8. Keep all of the tension firmly on the calf muscles as you lower your body.
9. Inhale for 2 seconds on the way down.
10. Do not bounce at any point of the exercise. Keep legs straight and knees and hips locked.

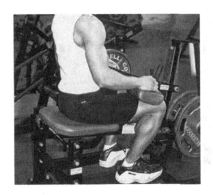 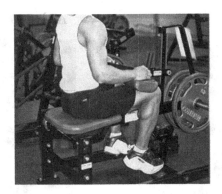

13. Seated Calf Raises

1. Sit on the seat with your knees under the pad and feet on the platform shoulder width apart with the balls of your feet on the platform and heels off.
2. Keep your torso erect, grasp the handles on top of the padding. Lock your hips and knees.
3. Keep your toes pointed forward and begin to tense your calf muscles.
4. Raise your heels as high as possible pushing the weight and padding up.
5. Focus on your calves performing all of the work when raising your lower legs up on the balls of your feet.
6. Exhale for 2 seconds on the way up.
7. Pause for 2 seconds at the top squeezing your calf muscles, contracting them fully.
8. Lower your heels as low as possible, below the platform until you feel a good stretch in your calves.
9. Inhale for 2 seconds on the way down.
10. Do not bounce at any point of the exercise, never using any momentum. Keep all of the tension on the calf muscles.

ABDOMINALS

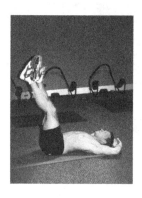 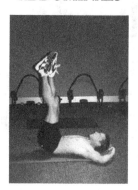

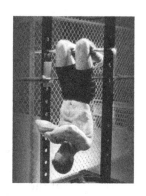 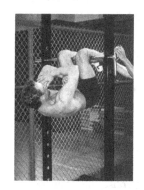

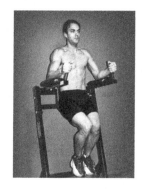 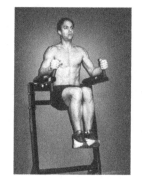

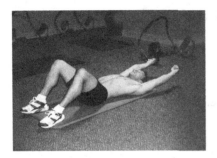 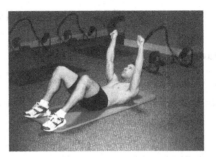

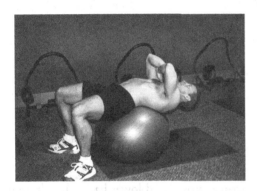 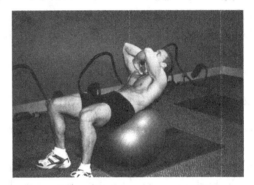

1. Each exercise included here for the abdominal region whether it be more focused on a certain region (upper/middle/lower/entire abs) or not is to be performed by the abs and no other parts of the body.
2. Whether it be leg raises (lower abs) or stability ball crunches (upper abs), you will use your abs only.
3. Beginning these exercises, you may want to place your hand on your abdominal section to get a feeling for what you are focusing on working in these exercises.
4. Maintain constant tension on your abs on the way up and down.
5. Maintain a slow, consistent rhythm under control (without bouncing or using momentum).
6. Exhale for 2 seconds on the way up.
7. Pause for 1 second at the top contracting your abs.
8. Inhale for 2 seconds on the way down.
9. With good focus in breathing and technique, your abs will feel the burn with a small number of repetitions (15-20). With a well balanced diet included, it won't be long before the desired ripples appear.
10. Keep the exercises basic. Switch them up from time to time and don't overdo them. Ultimately, a healthy diet will bring out all of the underlying work put forth from these exercises.

TOP TEN STRETCHES

1. Lying Hamstrings

1. Lie on the floor with knees bent.
2. Take a deep breath and relax your body from head to toe.
3. Straighten one leg and slowly pull it towards you.
4. Grab the top of your calf.
5. Keep knee slightly bent.
6. Bring the stretch to about a 6 on a 1-10 scale of pain.
7. You should feel the muscle stretch.
8. It should never feel like a pull or a sharp pain. If so, discontinue.
9. Hold for 10-15 seconds.
10. Switch and repeat using other leg.

2. Touch Floor, Touch Sky Stretch

1. Stand up tall with your feet shoulder width apart.
2. Keep a very slight bend in your knees.
3. Bend over from the waist and reach down as far as possible keeping legs straight.
4. Grab the back of your ankles and stretch your hamstrings, upper and lower back while keeping your head down.
5. Hold steady for 10-15 seconds.
6. You should feel a stretch, never a pain or a pull.
7. Rise to your starting/standing position.
8. Clasp your palms together.
9. Stretch your arms straight overhead as far as possible.
10. Hold for 10-15 seconds feeling the stretch in your upper body and arms.

3. Inner Thigh/Groin Stretch

1. Sit on the floor with your feet pressed together.
2. Keep abs in.
3. Draw your bellybutton in towards your spine.
4. Grab your ankles.
5. Place your elbows against the inside of your knees.
6. Lean forward from the waist.
7. Feel the gentle stretch in your inner thighs/groin area.
8. It should not be painful or feel like a pull.
9. To stretch farther, apply pressure on your inner knees with your elbows.
10. Hold for 10-15 seconds.

4. Lying Lower Back/Hips Stretch

1. Lie down on the floor.
2. Keep head and shoulders back.
3. Pull your knees into your chest.
4. Clasp your hands over your knees and upper chin.
5. Press your hips into the floor.
6. Focus on your low back and hips stretching.
7. Do not pull your knees too far in towards your chest. Upper body should stay on the floor.
8. The stretch should not hurt.
9. The stretch should not pull your lower back.
10. Hold for 10-15 seconds.

5. Lying Spinal Twist/Glute Stretch

1. Lie down on the floor.
2. Place your right foot on your left knee with your right leg bent across.
3. With your left hand, gently pull your right knee towards the floor.
4. Feel the stretch in your right glute muscle.
5. Gently twist your spine in the opposite direction.
6. Keep your left arm straight out.
7. Hips and shoulders should remain on the floor.
8. Do not stretch to the point of feeling pain.
9. Hold for 10-15 seconds.
10. Switch sides.

6. Seated Shoulder and Arms Stretch

1. This stretch can be done at your desk at work.
2. Sit up tall with good posture on your seat.
3. Interlace your fingers behind your back.
4. Palms should be facing your back.
5. Slowly turn your elbows inward.
6. Straighten your arms until a stretch is felt.
7. Lift your breast bone slightly upward as you stretch.
8. The stretch should not hurt.
9. The stretch should not pull at your shoulder joint.
10. Hold for 10-15 seconds.

7. Standing Back Stretch

1.   Stand with your feet shoulder width apart.
2.   Stand up tall.
3.   Keep a slight bend in your knees.
4.   Gently turn your torso at the waist.
5.   Look over your shoulder.
6.   You will feel your back stretching.
7.   Hold for 10-15 seconds.
8.   Remain steady in your stretch without any bouncing.
9.   Breathe normally (do not hold your breath).
10. Repeat on the other side.

8. Standing Chest Stretch

1.   Stand in a doorway with your feet shoulder width apart.
2.   Place your right forearm on the side of the doorway wall at chest level.
3.   Keep your elbow bent at 90 degrees.
4.   Slowly turn your body to the left.
5.   Focus on your chest muscle.
6.   You should feel a nice stretch through the right side of your chest.
7.   Do not turn your body too far.
8.   It should not hurt in your shoulder joint.
9.   Hold consistently for 10-15 seconds.
10. Switch sides and repeat.

9. Standing Quadricep Stretch

1.   Stand with your feet shoulder width apart and hold onto a wall for balance.
2.   Take your right leg off of the ground.
3.   Grab the top of your right foot and bend your knee.
4.   Gently bring the foot towards your buttocks.
5.   Keep your knee pointed straight at the floor.
6.   You should feel the stretch right down the quadricep.
7.   You can squeeze your hips forward to feel more of a stretch in the hip flexors.
8.   Hold for 10-15 seconds.
9.   Do not bounce or pull your feet too far back.
10. Switch sides and repeat.

10. Tricep Stretch

1. Stand with your feet shoulder width apart.
2. Stand with good posture.
3. Bend your left elbow behind your head.
4. Use your right hand to gently pull your left elbow in.
5. You should feel a stretch in your tricep. Left palm touching your back.
6. Do not move your shoulder as this will take away from the stretch.
7. Hold steady and do not bounce.
8. Do not pull your elbow too far back.
9. Hold for 10-15 seconds.
10. Switch sides and repeat.

CHAPTER 6

SUPER HEALTH PROGRAMS FOR PROFESSIONS M-Z

	Activity Level	Stress Level
	6.5	3.5

11. MANUFACTURING & PRODUCTION 🏭

It's part of the job!

At work, you are on your feet most of the day. The work that you perform daily can become monotonous and it can be hard to stay motivated throughout the day. Once you get in a daily routine and understand the procedures at your job, mental challenges may be deficient. As a result, this can lead to complacency and a development of lackadaisical habits. This can negatively impact your physical health, as well as your overall well being.

The work can become physical at times forcing you to put your body in awkward, compromising positions. You are around machinery often, so you must be aware, alert, and on your toes. There is a possibility that you can get injured if you are not attentive because machines, like humans, are imperfect.

10. *Lifestyle Tips*

Be aware of your surroundings at work! It can become easy to fall into the proverbial rut and be surrounded by negative attitudes. Take advantage of your breaks. Get outside and take in some healthy air for a while. Try to limit/avoid smoke environments and also consuming too much caffeine. Since you will be on your feet most of the day working, wear comfortable, supporting shoes.

Set some daily/weekly goals to achieve. You know when you are working and when you are not (7-3, 3-11, 11-7, etc.) so plan your daily schedule in advance to achieve some goals. You will be amazed at how much you can get accomplished with good planning. Who knows? You may choose to go to (back to) college to stimulate your mind. Don't become lazy and complacent. Keep the fire burning brightly! Have something to look forward to that will keep you motivated and this will make your days much happier.

9. *All-Star Foods and Liquid Fuel* (■ all TOP TEN FIT FAST FOODS)

Most factories and shops usually have a set shift with set hours for a 45 min-1 hour lunch break and a couple of short breaks during the day. There isn't any reason why you shouldn't be eating your way to SUPER HEALTH.

FOODS AT WORK

➤ Apples, pears, raspberries, strawberries, oranges (rich in vitamin C-which is a must, especially in a smoke environment)
➤ Low-fat cottage cheese (rich in amino acids & is a complete protein)
➤ Grinders/hoagies on wheat (low-fat choices-6/8 grams of fat)
➤ Multi-grain bread w/ oven roasted turkey breast (4-6 oz) w/ hot sauce, tomato salad

SNACKS AT WORK

➤ Clif bars, Luna bars, Kashi Go-Lean bars, low-fat yogurt, Polly-O string-ums lite mozzarella sticks, Pure Protein bars

FOODS AT HOME

➤ Old-fashioned oatmeal, 3 egg whites, 1 egg yolk, orange juice, grapefruit
➤ Shrimp salad w/ olive oil & vinegar, roasted asparagus, couscous
➤ Roasted duck/chicken breast, whole wheat pasta, celery sticks, cucumber salad
➤ Top round sirloin steak, three bean salad, sweet potato/yam
➤ Salmon (4-6 oz.), brown rice, roasted eggplant, steamed mixed veggies

Liquid Fuel

• Consume 120 oz. water daily. Have it by your station. If you aren't able to do this, drink 20 oz. water every break.
• Keep caffeinated beverages to a minimum (0-1 a day)

8. *Foods to Avoid*

➤ Vending machine snacks: chips, cookies, crackers, pretzels, granola bars, soda, chocolate
➤ Deli grinders: w/ pastrami, ham, roast beef, corn beef, bologna w/ mayo & cheese
  • Note: These cold cuts are high in fat and sodium, 2 SUPER HEALTH killers!

> ➤ Lasagna, ravioli, gnocchi, chicken parmigiana, eggplant parmigiana, shrimp alfredo
> ➤ Other quick hits: donuts, danishes, croissants, muffins, bagels, cappuccino, light & sweet coffee, hot chocolate
> ➤ Burritos, tacos, grilled cheese sandwich
> ➤ General Tsao's chicken, fried white rice, egg rolls
> ➤ Pork chops, veal, sausage, bacon
> ➤ High sugar breakfast cereals w/ whole milk
> ➤ Alcoholic beverages (limit 1-3 glasses of wine weekly)
> ➤ Pizza

7. Meals: How many & when?

Throughout the workday, your body requires a sufficient amount of sustained energy. To accomplish this, you must consume more meals (approx. every 3 hours) while working than while being at home.

<u>Here's the breakdown:</u> (ex. for a 7-3 shift)

6 A.M.	breakfast
9 A.M.	all-star snack
12 P.M.	medium-sized lunch
3 P.M.	small all-star meal
6 P.M.	dinner

6. Supplementation & Sleep

We profess a consistent sleep of 7-8 hours a night all week. Avoid skipping an hour or two each day during the workweek and then sleeping in to "catch up" during the weekend. There is no such thing as "catching up". Get your weekend days started on the right track by hitting the gym in the morning.

During the week, you can take a 10-minute power nap after work and before resistance training to recharge your batteries.

What supplements are right for you?
   <u>A List</u>

1. multivitamin
2. antioxidants- help fight free radicals, which may be abundant due to poorer air quality at work (high in vitamin C & E)

3. meal replacements

4. vitamin C (extra 1000 mg. daily)

<u>B List</u>

1. echinacea

2. vitamin B (100 mg)

3. melatonin

4. caffeine (200 mg. before training)-should be only time taken

5. tyrosine

5. *Resistance Training* (📖 TOP TEN TOPICS, proper form)

- Four days: 2 days during week & 2 times on the weekend

Workouts on the weekend:

- You will be rested and have more energy to hit the gym
- 1 hour on Saturday, 1 hour on Sunday, in the morning
- Endorphins produced during workout will get you in the right frame of mind for the weekend

Workouts during the workweek:

- Train Tuesday & Thursday after work (& after a 10 minute powernap)

A workout right for you!
- FEMALES: 3 sets/exercise, 12-15 reps, 75-85% failure
- MALES: 3 sets/exercise, 8-10 reps; 80-90% failure

<u>UPPER BODY</u> **Tuesday & Saturday**

- **Use exercises that recruit primary & secondary muscles.**
- **Standing exercises are preferable.**

  2) Warm up w/ 50 pushups (or less depending on strength levels)
  3) Standing cable crossover (cables)
  NOTE: Line up the cable pulley w/ the middle of your chest
  4) Pull ups (use assisted machine if necessary)
  5) Standing bicep curls
  6) Standing tricep extensions
  7) Standing dumbbell shoulder press

8) Standing dumbbell lateral raises
9) Low back extension machine
10) Hanging leg raises

LOWER BODY Thursday & Sunday

- **These exercises will recruit muscle fibers into action.**
- **Standing exercises are preferable.**

1) Warm up w/ 100 jumping jacks
2) Squats*
NOTE: Perform a leg press as an alternate if not comfortable, have weak knees/low back or don't have a spotter
3) Stiff leg dead lifts*
NOTE: Perform a lying leg curl as an alternate
4) Standing calf raises
5) 100 jumping jacks
6) Stability ball crunches

*These are high-risk exercises that should be performed w/ a partner paying careful attention to proper form.

HOT BODYPARTS
$$$ LOW BACK $$$

Standing all day on the job requires a strong lower back for support. Maintain good form while performing all of your exercises. In addition to strengthening your lower back, the exercises provided will strengthen your inner core muscles (within the abdominal cavity).

4. *Cardiovascular training*
    ❑ **3 days a week of mind-clearing cardio is a big stress reliever**

TUESDAY

- After weight training for 21 minutes

TYPE	TIME	INTENSITY	HR
1) INTERVAL CYCLING	5 min.	slow	(60-65%)
	2 min.	fast	(80-85%)

Alternate between these two intensities for 21 minutes.

THURSDAY

- After weight training for 21 minutes

TYPE	*TIME*	*INTENSITY*	*HR*
1) INTERVAL STEPMILL	5 min.-	slow	(60-70%)
	2 min.	fast	(80-90%)

Alternate between these two intensities for 21 minutes.

SATURDAY or SUNDAY

- 30 minutes
- Take a jog or bicycle (preferably outdoors-enjoy the fresh air)

For the ambitious minded:
**During the workweek, go outside on your lunch break and take a nice 30-45 min. brisk walk.

3. *Sports*
Enjoy some relaxing, yet friendly competitive sports

- Company softball league
- Bowling league
- Company golf league
- Basketball
- Racquetball

2. *How to Move More*   <u>Activity level</u>   <u>6.5</u>

In this field, you are forced to be on the move most of the time. Although you may not be lifting strenuous equipment all of the time, intermittently you are probably lifting, throwing, squatting, reaching, pushing, and/or pulling various items.

Whether you are standing, sitting, or moving around all day, be certain to check your posture. Keep your chest up and shoulders back. This will save on your lower back, which is being strengthened in your weight training.

Get out of a stagnant atmosphere to enjoy some fresh circulating air. Also, while at work on a break, find an open area and perform 20-30 pushups.

1. *Obstacles and Ways To Conquer Them*

1. Staying motivated in a not-so motivating environment

Rise above it all! Don't settle for mediocrity. Use the "Top 10 Tools" on a daily basis. Join the company's leagues and become a leader. Get outside as much as possible. Take control of your life. Go back to school and take advantage of the opportunities out there. You have 8 hours a day during the week to dedicate towards other attainable goals.

2. Avoiding bad habits

Countless cups of coffee, smoking, laziness, and poor eating, are habits that you may very well observe at your workplace amongst people. Research has shown that it takes 3-4 weeks of consistent daily repetition to create a habit (both good and bad). Realizing this fact, wake up everyday and make it a goal to challenge your inner self to eat well and workout in the gym. We realize that initially it will be hard, but what doesn't kill you, makes you stronger in the end!

3. Work is monotonous & not mentally challenging/stimulating

You may feel as if you are a robot because you perform the same tasks day in and day out. You may feel that your work is not being appreciated. If you bring a great work ethic to the table everyday, it will eventually get noticed. We guarantee it!

	Activity Level	Stress Level
	1.5	5.5

12. PINK COLLAR EMPLOYEES 📖

It's part of the job!

The "working woman" is what you are in more ways than one or two for that matter! You have the responsibility of the world weighted on your shoulders (or at least it feels like that at times). Waking up in the morning and making sure the children are prepared for school and then off they go, followed by a full-work day on your part, to then return home to take care of the family and all of their "needs" & "wants". Lastly, you will go to bed at night to wake up and do it all over again in another "unique" form. It is quite an interesting compilation of daily challenges & responsibilities that you must take on.

If we simply focus on your time at work, then that may be enough for you already. You have to endure different people's problems and come up with solutions to solve them. Maybe you have to deal with a boss or co-workers on a daily basis that you truly would rather not be around. That can raise the stress level up just a notch or two. Let's not talk about what is awaiting you when you return home for the evening and you hear voices asking, "What's for dinner?"

Your activity level throughout the day is low. Consequently, this sedentary state warrants the fat molecules that we consume to settle most happily and readily in our body. Being inside an office facility all day does not facilitate active, long-distance ventures on a regular basis. You are busy making decisions and plans interacting with many people all day long.

10. *Lifestyle Tips*

Find a reason, any reason to MOVE, MOVE, & MOVE SOME MORE! This is vital to your wellness because your time is sparse throughout the course of a day, so finding any reason to move at work will keep your body chugging and burning those calories.

Bring your all-star foods with you on a regular basis to prevent from binging on any other foods that "don't make the cut"!

Work out right before or after work. You make the call which time frame is the more doable of the two. Once you've made the call, stick to it! This will aid in your time management and you'll have something to look forward to on a daily basis. Your energy levels will be higher and spirits rising higher than ever, which will greatly enhance all aspects of your life. Spring board your way to SUPER HEALTH!

A QUICK REVIEW ON YOUR LIFESTYLE TIPS:

MOVE, MOVE, MOVE SOME MORE!!!!!!!!! (just in case you forgot)

9. All-Star Foods and Liquid Fuel

FOODS AT WORK (bring your food with you)

➤ **High-fiber grains & cereals** (use the 5/5 cereal rule-less than 5 grams of sugar, more than/at least 5 grams of fiber): ex. all-bran cereals, Fiberone, Grapenuts, Shredded Wheat
➤ **More high fiber foods:** leafy vegetables & salads (w/ olive oil & vinegar w/ grilled chicken breast), broccoli, carrots, oatmeal, barley
  • Fiber takes longer to chew so you won't be tempted to overeat.
  • Your body utilizes more calories to break down high fiber foods, which in turn elevates your metabolism.
  • This is very beneficial for your particular daily routine.
➤ **High protein foods:** grilled chicken breast, hard-boiled eggs w/out the yolk, tuna fish, low-fat yogurt, cottage cheese, Polly-O-stringum lite mozzarella sticks, veggie burgers, soymilk
➤ **Berries:** strawberries, raspberries, blueberries
  • These help balance hormones.
  • These help prevent menstrual cramping.
  • These reduce the development of varicose veins.

FOODS AT HOME

➤ **Low-glycemic carbohydrates:** (these include your high-fiber choices) soybeans (high in phytoe-strogens), chickpeas, sweet potatoes, yams, couscous, baked beans
➤ **Egg white omelette** w/ peppers, spinach, tomatoes, hot sauce (metabolism booster), orange juice, grapefruit, rye toast
➤ **Fish:** trout, oysters, swordfish, salmon, halibut, cod, shrimp w/ brown rice & mixed steam veggies
➤ **Other favorites:**
  • Top round steak (4 oz.), green beans, coleslaw, mushroom
  • Basil rotini tomato soup, 99% fat-free chicken noodle soup, tofu products, cobb salad, cucumber salad, deli pickles, three-bean salads

HOT TIP
#1

*Ladies, stay disciplined with your diet 90-95% of the month and when you are premenstrual, then you are allowed to indulge in what you crave. This once a month binge will not hurt you if you otherwise stay consistent.

OUR PERSONAL RECOMMENDED INDULGENCE CHOCOLATE BAR:

Dove dark chocolate bar!

<u>*Liquid Fuel*</u>

- Water (120 oz. daily)
- Decaffeinated beverages (ex. green tea)

8. Foods to Avoid

High sugar foods

chips	fat-free snacks (most are high in sugar)
chocolate	cookies
ice cream	chocolate donuts
frozen yogurt	chocolate muffins
sorbet	chocolate milkshake

High trans fat foods

high-fat salad dressing	frozen entrees
non-dairy creamers	processed dinner aids
processed foods	pre-made dips
hydrogenated oil products (a.k.a. trans fat)	

High GI foods

pretzels	cornflakes
jellybeans	donuts
French bread	chocolate
breads	rice cakes

(on label of bread product, if the 1st ingredient is unbleached flour, put it back on the shelf)

High fat meals (high calorie)

eggplant parmigiana	chicken parmigiana
nachos & cheese	pizza
gnocchis	macaroni & cheese
dark turkey meat, stuffing, biscuits	
bacon, egg, & cheese on a bagel/roll	

HOT TIP
#1

*Cook with olive oil or other oils high in monounsaturated fats (ex. flaxseed oil).

#2

*Bake, broil, grill, or boil the meals for your family.

<u>Caffeinated beverages</u>

What role does caffeine have with calcium?

 ➢   Caffeine limits the calcium availability in your body and can result in further loss of calcium over time.

7. Meals: How many & when?
    Your goal is to consume 5 small meals a day. This routine will keep your insulin levels and blood sugar levels more stable by consuming frequent small carb/moderate protein meals. This is just what you need for tackling a "full-day's plate" of activities. Try and eat the same amount of calories with each meal. You MUST eat upon waking up to get the metabolism going. DO NOT SKIP BREAKFAST! Antagonistically speaking, do not eat past 8 P.M.

6. Supplementation & Sleep
    Sleep 7-8 hours a night consistently. If you keep yourself busy & active throughout the day by working out regularly, moving as much as possible at work & going home and spending quality time with your family, then your body will be ready to take on the sleep it so deserves.

What supplements are right for you?
    <u>A List</u>

        1. multivitamin & multimineral
        2. antioxidant
        3. calcium (1000 mg)
        4. EFAs

    <u>B List</u>

        1. CLA
        2. ginseng & ginkgo

5. *Resistance Training* (📖 TOP TEN TOPICS, does lifting weights build muscles in women)
- WHEN: Three days a week (Mon/Wed/Fri)
- TIME: Immediately before or after work (consistently)
- TYPE: Circuit training
  - 15 repetitions/exercise, 3 total circuits
  - 10-20 second rest in between exercises
  - 2 minute rest between circuits
  - HR should be above 55% throughout the workout

A workout right for you!

CIRCUIT #1

- ***Total body workout that will get you moving, grooving, & losing those pounds!***

  · Body weight squats
  · Leg extensions
  · Lying leg curls
  · Dumbbell chest press
  · Machine shoulder press
  · Standing tricep extensions
  · Standing bicep curls
  · Abdominal crunches/stability ball
  · Lat rows

CIRCUIT #2

REPEAT CIRCUIT #1

CIRCUIT #3

REPEAT CIRCUIT #1

4. *Cardiovascular training*
  - ❏ 3 days a week (MON/WED/FRI), 15-20 minutes after resistance training
  - ❏ MON-Stairmaster; WED-Elliptical X-trainer; FRI-Treadmill
  - ❏ Use this alternating sequence:

TIME	INTENSITY	HEART RATE
3 min	slow & easy	60-70%
2 min	fast & hard	75-85%

On TUESDAY or THURSDAY:

❖ First thing in the morning, do 45 minutes of cardio at 65-75% HR (fitness level-dependent). This will be great for fat catabolism. Your body will use more fat for energy.
  - **Fat-burning results can be maximized by waiting 1-hour to eat following completion of your cardio session. These effects work for solo cardio sessions (not combined with resistance training).**
  - **For you go-getter independent-minded working women, do cardio on BOTH Tuesday and Thursday for ultimate fitness.**

NOTE: The elliptical x-trainer is a non-impact low stress machine on your joints and also works the upper body as well as the lower body simultaneously. This will boost the amount of calories that you burn in a session.

3. *Sports*
Enjoy some breathtaking activities to keep you moving

  - Tennis
  - Gardening (220 cal/hour burned)
  - Yoga/Pilates (1 day a week)
  - Hiking (480 cal/hr burned)
  - Golf (use a golf stroller to carry your clubs vs. a cart-you will burn an extra 320 calories this way and take in some clean fresh air better)
  - rollerblading

2. *How to Move More*   <u>Activity level</u>   <u>1.5</u> (📖 TOP TEN TOPICS, calories a person burns daily)

This section of tips pertaining to your professional field is one that you need to listen to carefully. Your overall activity level throughout the day is very low. It is important that you follow the tips that we outline for you in this customized program to break the vicious cycle of low-to-no movement throughout the day. We have recommended top tips for you to implement both at work and at home.

Top Tips for "Ms. Independent" (at work)

  - Every hour you must get up and move. Remind yourself with an alarm clock.

TIME*	MOVEMENT*
10 A.M.	Stand up, stretch arms to ceiling, hold for 10 seconds, stretch arms down to floor, keep legs straight, hold for 10 seconds

11 A.M.	Get up and go to the bathroom and take the stairs
12 P.M. (lunch)	Go outside and walk
1 P.M.	Go to the bathroom again and take the long way
2 P.M.	50 small arm circles to the front while standing up
3 P.M.	50 small arm circles to the rear while standing up
4 P.M.	Repeat 10 A.M. movement

*This is one example of many. You can switch the exercises and hours from time to time.

- Sit with good posture at all times (chest up, abs tight)
- Drink water throughout the day reaping all of its benefits (this will force you to GET UP, MOVE AGAIN and hit the ladies room)
- Listen to upbeat music at work (when you can)
- Fidget (people who fidget on a daily basis burn an extra 150 calories a day)

Top Tips for "half" Woman & "half" Amazing
(at home)

- Stay active by getting involved in family activities during the weekends (check out "Sports" section).
- Sitting in front of the tube for the night may not be your best bet. Get up during commercials to move about. Fidget while you watch television.
- Take the stairs whenever possible.
- Park a distance away from stores.

1. *Obstacles and Ways To Conquer Them*

1. Staying active/on track at work when you may not feel well

The key message here is consistency. If you are consistent with your exercising routines, eating habits, & sleep habits for 90-95% of the time, who could ask for anything more? You will have that time during the month when your body craves something delicious & sweet. We recommend that you indulge & satisfy your body's cravings. But remember, get right back on track and get "consistent" again. You can afford those slack days at work by having a diet that is consistent throughout (as the overriding driving force)!

2. Heavy workloads halting your motivation to continue working out

Small changes for the better each day turn in to big changes in the future. Trust us when we say that you can do it. You may even surprise yourself, but you can achieve whatever your mind believes to be true. Use your "Top 10 Tools". Separate work from home. Drink a cup of coffee in the morning if you need that kickstart (just before hitting the gym). Just drink extra water & add another calcium supplement to your diet. Set the bar high for yourself at work and you will be more inclined to stick to other goals outside of work as well.

3. Keeping a smile on your face & pleasing your boss

Exercising regularly releases valuable chemicals which can promote a natural euphoric state of mind. Stick with it and when you witness your own results first hand, then that smile will light up more than your boss's face. Speak to your husband about what we mean!

Activity Level	Stress Level
5.5	3.5

13. RETAIL & GROCERY ☺

It's part of the job!

During the course of your day, your feet will let you know how they feel. Whether you are stocking shelves, moving boxes, pulling and pushing carriages, bagging groceries, checking people out as a cashier, you spend quite a bit of time on your feet. Much of that time spent on your feet is hard work.

You deal with a constant influx of different people throughout the day. These people may have questions, comments, and concerns that are expressed to you. You need to possess extremely good customer service skills in dealing with the general public. People make the difference in a business. The attitude that you bring forth with you to work can dictate whether customers will return or find somewhere else to go for business.

10. *Lifestyle Tips*

Due to the fact that you are standing on your feet for a good majority of the day, make sure that you stand with good posture and wear comfortable shoes that support your lower back.

Plan to workout in the morning so you will be burning calories at an elevated rate throughout the day. Your energy levels will be sky high and you will be in the right frame of mind to keep that smile on all day long.

As the day progresses, eat downhill. Consume the most calories during the morning and the least amount of calories at night.

You utilize many muscle groups throughout the day including your legs, back, arms, and shoulders. These should be your primary focus areas for strengthening on a weekly basis.

Set goals for yourself! Many of the positions in this profession are either part-time or low-income. If you enjoy your job, that's great! Then, you may want to set your sights at trying to move up in the company/store or go back to school and further your life-long learning.

9. *All-Star Foods and Liquid Fuel* (☺ all TOP TEN FIT FAST FOODS)

FOODS AT WORK

➤ Dried fruits (raisins, prunes, apples, apricots, nectarines)
➤ Sunflower seeds, almonds, Brazil nuts
➤ Canned tuna fish (albacore) w/ rye bread, deli pickle
➤ Subway (grilled chicken breast w/ wheat bread, no cheese, hot sauce, red & green peppers, lettuce, tomato)

➢ Meal replacements & banana, Clif bar, Luna bar, Pure Protein bar
➢ Carrot sticks, cucumbers, celery sticks, chicken soup, hard-boiled eggs, low-fat yogurt

FOODS AT HOME

➢ 4 egg white omelette w/ tomatoes, broccoli, beans, low-fat cheddar cheese, orange juice, 1 slice multi-grain toast
➢ Grilled chicken breast w/ hot sauce, brown rice, corn on the cob
➢ Ground lean turkey meat, split pea soup, baked beans, cucumber salad
➢ Oatmeal, Kashi Go-Lean cereal w/ 1% milk/Fiberone, Grapenuts w/ soymilk
➢ Lean cuts of meat (top-round, sirloin, flank) w/ mixed veggies, sweet potato

HOT TIP:
#1

*Grocery workers: spend time and shop in the produce and natural food sections. This is where most of your all-star food choices are found.

Liquid Fuel

• Caffeine in moderation (1 cup-morning)
• 16 oz. sports water bottle within arms reach all of the time, fill up & drink 6 a day
• green tea (decaffeinated)
• limit alcohol consumption (treat yourself once a week)

8. Foods to Avoid

GROCERY STORE WORKERS:

It is easier for you to choose the all-star food choices and stay clear of the foods to avoid than it is for people at other jobs.

➢ Deli
  • Stay away from the luncheon meats, as most are high in sodium and highly processed.
  • Avoid the fried products in the hot case.

HOT TIP:

#1

*Many deli foods are high in sodium & fat (which is not mentioned on the label). This means that if these products are consumed often, then you will have to supplement with an increased water intake and additional movement to burn the excess calories.

- ➤ **Frozen foods section**
  - With the exception of vegetables, try to avoid this section.
- ➤ **Dairy section**
  - Whole milk
  - Cheeses
- ➤ **Bakery**
  - Cakes
  - Cookies
  - Donuts
  - Muffins
  - Croissants
  - White-flour breads (bagels, Portuguese rolls, hoagie rolls, sandwich rolls)

RETAILERS

- ➤ **Take out foods all of the time**
  - Pizza
  - Chinese
  - Fast foods (not from our "fit-fast food" section)

- ➤ **Refined sugars**
  - White rice
  - High-sugar cereals
  - Fruit juices
  - Sports drinks
  - Soda
  - Caffeinated beverages/alcoholic beverages in excess
  - Vending machine foods

7. Meals: How many & when?

Throughout the workday, your body's metabolism will be slowing down. With that in mind, breakfast should be your largest meal for two reasons. First, it gives you the energy necessary for an optimal day at work. Secondly, your body is at its highest metabolic rate upon awakening so that is when the calories are burned the quickest. As the day progresses, each meal should progressively get smaller. In between breakfast, lunch, and dinner you should consume some small all-star snacks.

<u>Here's the breakdown:</u> (ex. for a 7-3 shift)

6 A.M.	breakfast (most calories for a meal)
9 A.M.	small all-star snack
12 P.M.	medium-sized lunch
3 P.M.	small all-star snack
6 P.M.	small dinner (least calories for a meal)

6. Supplementation & Sleep

Get in the habit of obtaining 7-8 hours of sleep daily. This will set you up for an incredibly energized workweek.

What supplements are right for you?

<u>A List</u>

1. multivitamin
2. antioxidant

<u>B List</u>

1. glucosamine/chondroitin
2. tyrosine
3. melatonin
4. ZMA

5. Resistance Training

- Three days: Monday, Wednesday, Friday (in the morning)
- Workout 30 minutes after waking up
- Drink ½ meal replacement + a fruit upon awakening
- Drink other ½ of meal replacement right after training
- Eat breakfast within an hour of workout

<u>3 day splits</u>
- ➤ Monday- push routine (chest, triceps, shoulders)
- ➤ Wednesday- pull routine (back, biceps)
- ➤ Friday- legs, abs

A workout right for you!
- FEMALES: 3 sets/exercise, 12-15 reps, 75-89% failure on last 2 reps
- MALES: 3 sets/exercise, 8-10 reps; 90-99% failure on last 2 reps
- 1-1.5 minute rest in between sets and exercises.

HOT TIP:
#1

*You have to continue to overload your muscles to overcome challenges.

<u>MONDAY</u> (PUSH)

1) Dumbbell incline press
2) Standing tricep extensions with straight bar
3) Seated dumbbell shoulder press
4) Side lateral raises
5) Flat bench press
6) 30-50 pushups (advanced=try handstand pushups)- only 1 set

HOT EXERCISE:

<u>HANDSTAND PUSHUPS</u>

Stand on your hands with your heels on the wall and perform as many handstand pushups as possible. Push your body and arms straight up, then your entire body and head will be approaching ½ inch close to the ground. This is a very challenging exercise that will develop great upper body strength.

<u>WEDNESDAY</u> (PULL)

1) Pull ups (use assisted machine if needed)
2) Seated lat rows
3) Machine preacher curls
4) Standing barbell curls
5) Seated hammer curls
6) Low back extensions on 45 deg. bench (hold weight on your chest to challenge yourself)

<u>FRIDAY</u> (LEGS, ABS)

1) Squats
2) Lying leg curls
3) Seated leg curls
4) Leg extensions
5) Standing calf raises
6) Hanging leg raises (3 sets/20 reps)
7) Stability ball crunches (3 sets/20 reps)

HOT TIP:
#1

*Hold your arms straight over your head on the stability ball crunches for a more challenging alternative.

HOT BODY PARTS
$$$ ARMS & SHOULDERS $$$

Moving things around all day require some serious muscular strength & endurance in your arms & shoulders. While in the gym, focus on these muscles, taking the exercises slow and burning out those bi's, tri's, & shoulders.

4. *Cardiovascular training* (☺ TOP TEN TOPICS, high vs. low intense cardio)
   - ❏ **3 days a week- for 20 minutes after resistance training**
   - ❏ **Maintain heart rate at 75-85%**
   - ❏ **Choose from the following exercises:**
     1) **stationary bike**
     2) **stairmaster**
     3) **elliptical x-trainer**
     4) **stepmill**

Choose either Tuesday or Thursday to do 45 minutes of low-intense cardio in the morning.

3. *Sports*

Your hours at work may require you to work at night, during some holidays, on the weekends, or even (on rare occasions, hopefully) some double shifts. Despite that fact, you should still get 2 days off during the week. This time can be spent enjoying some fun, sporting activities that are a good outlet for relieving the stresses from the workweek.

Enjoy some great stress-relieving activities

- Spinning classes (good choice to get you off of your feet)
- Mountain biking
- Rowing, kayaking
- Ice skating
- Cross-country skiing (you will be using muscles from all over your body)

2. *How to Move More*   <u>Activity level</u>   <u>5.5</u>

You are on your feet constantly at work so your activity level is fairly high. Stretch your hamstrings & low back on the hour. Tight hamstrings can lead to a tight low back. Throughout the days, weeks, & months, the repetitive motions that your body endures at work can take a toll on you, resulting in possible back injuries if you are not careful. Again, stretch each hour, bending over at the waist. Touch your toes or the floor (if possible) and hold for 15 seconds (without bouncing) keeping a slight bend in your knees.

If you are a stockperson:

- Lift with your legs. Keep chest up & abs tight.
- Be careful when stocking items over your head.

If you are more customer service-oriented:

- Keep a smile on first and foremost.
- Stand with good posture.
- Take your breaks & lunch outside to get some fresh air (if possible).

1. *Obstacles and Ways To Conquer Them*

1. Hitting goals	Set monthly, weekly, daily goals for yourself. Do not stop until you obtain them. If you are a part-time employee, set the goal to be full-time, maybe even a manager. Why stop there? How about becoming district manager? Set high standards for yourself at the workplace and this will translate to your work ethic in other areas of your life that relate to SUPER HEALTH!
2. Time management	If you are a full-time student during the day and work at night or in some cases two jobs due to income needs, then you have to

be extremely disciplined with your time & how you use it. If you don't think that it's possible, sit down and take some notes on where your time is spent throughout the day. From there, you can plan better to spend 5 out of 112 waking hours training and maybe 2 hours preparing some all-star foods. In the long run, there isn't anything more valuable than that time well spent!

3. Staying positive & motivated around people all day

Eating properly will help maintain your blood sugar level during the day. Exercising frequently will keep your spirits rising high. Combine these two factors and you end up with a smile that comes natural. Your boss will notice the value of that smile soar through the roof!

4. Using your arms at work a lot

Hit those hot body parts in the gym & don't be afraid to hit them HARD!

5. Good eating patterns

Eating downhill throughout the day is a must! Eating sound nutritionally is 80% of SUPER HEALTH! The energy lift that your body will have for most of the day will be that much better.

Activity Level	Stress Level
3.5	5.0

14. RIGHT-SIDE OF THE BRAIN THINKERS ❧

It's part of the job!

You see the answers to many problems from different perspectives that may not be so obvious to others. You are a creator and highly intelligent in your practice. Many times, you may sit for extended hours engrossed in your work without realizing the time. Some of you spend much of your work time alone, while others of you work in groups to study, analyze, and research data. You may be looking at a computer screen, charts, graphs, and various literatures all day. There are also times when you are outdoors with your work, hopefully enjoying the natural world.

10. *Lifestyle Tips*

You may be sitting and spending quite a bit of time by yourself. Being your own boss allows a lot of leeway. Stay disciplined and motivated in your lifestyle by simply finding ways to move more and eat less throughout the day. Eating less does not mean cutting out a meal. Actually, you should be certain to eat small meals frequently.

If you are self-employed, try working where the environment is pleasant. Outdoors in a natural setting near the water or the trees can be a great venue for your mind to run wild with creativity. The tranquil, placid environment can relieve accumulated stresses built up due to deadlines, heavy workloads, or pressure to satisfy monetary necessities. If you are in a seated position for a long time, sit with good posture (shoulders back and chest up-your back will thank you later).

9. *All-Star Foods and Liquid Fuel*

Low GI carbohydrates

*These low glycemic carbs will increase your physical & mental longevity throughout the day. Your body requires a constant flow of glucose to fuel the brain for optimal work performance.

bran flakes	Kashi Go-Lean cereal
Fiber one cereal	whole wheat pasta
shredded wheat	old-fashioned oatmeal
sweet potatoes (high in antioxidants)	

Low-GI meat alternatives

garden burger
veggie burger
soy burger

Low-fat meat

sirloin	lean pork
top round	venison
flank	chicken/turkey breast

Low-fat products

fat-free cottage cheese
couscous
milk (low-fat)
soymilk
cheese (low-fat)

Healthy snacks by your work station

protein bars	apple
soy nuts	carrot sticks
yogurt	sunflower seeds

Quality high protein meals

1) albacore tuna on rye (made w/ low-fat mayo)
2) turkey breast, veggie cheese on pumpernickel
3) grilled chicken breast on wheat pita
4) 4 egg white omelette w/ spinach, mushroom, red pepper, hot sauce
5) fish (shrimp, sushi, shellfish-ex. oysters, mussels, clams) w/ brown rice
   NOTE: This is the "ultimate brain food" that will help fuel the right side of your brain.

<u>Additional all-star foods</u>

barley	leafy greens
English muffin	steamed veggies
apple butter	corn
pickles	

Liquid Fuel

Always have water by your side!! Get a 20 oz. bottle and fill it up 5 times a day (=100 oz)

Additional goodie: -GREEN TEA (hot or cold) or other caffeine-free herbal teas (instead of coffee)

-GRAPE JUICE (w/ breakfast)

HOT TIP:
#1

*Cook with monounsaturated oils (olive, canola, peanut, flax).

8. Foods to Avoid

If you are in a fixed position for a long period of time, it is very important to avoid any food or drink that gives you a quick burst of energy.

A) <u>High GI foods</u>

donuts	cookies
bagels	muffins
high-sugar cereals + whole milk	biscuits
scones	white refined flours
icc cream	(ex. enriched foods-white bread/pasta)
soda	milkshakes
café mochas/lattes	

HOT TIP
#1

*Stay disciplined around the holidays by reducing the portions of your actual meals.

B) Processed foods

Fast food, canned foods, frozen foods (high in sodium & fat)

C) Foods high in saturated fat

butter	corn oil
cheese	pork
bacon	sausage
fried chicken	French fries

D) Foods high in hydrogenated oils

margarine	crackers
wheat thins	cream substitutes
macaroni & cheese	shortening
stuffing mix	cream cheese

HOT TIP
#1

*Check the ingredients on many foods. Foods that you may think are all right to eat due to their low-fat content may have some of these "hazardous" oils in them.

7. Meals: How many & when?

Your biggest meal of the day should be breakfast. Following this meal, eat a small "high protein/ medium carb" (Low GI) meal. This will give you a steady flow of glucose (energy) throughout the day, which is necessary for mental processes to be functioning optimally. Your mind is your asset and you want to keep it that way. Your spatial/creative side needs to be fed fuel for maximum productivity.

When you are working, you may find yourself engulfed in whatever project it is that you are doing. To remind your body that it's time to eat, have a beeper, alarm clock, or a watch near by to go off indicating that it is time to eat.

6. *Supplementation & Sleep*

For many of you, you are your own boss. Therefore, you have the power to set your time clock. Don't let breakfast be at 12:00 P.M. Get energized early on for a complete day of success. You should be obtaining 7-8 hours of sleep a night on a consistent basis.

As we stated prior, you may get "in the zone" as you work and lose track of time. Try taking a 10-15 minute powernap mid-afternoon to recharge your mental and physical batteries. The medium that you are working with whether it be a canvas, a house, a building, clay, you need to have a clear picture in your mind on what it is that you intend to achieve. Often times, with a clear mind, it takes sufficient time. Stay consistent with your sleeping patterns and "the million dollar idea" for success may come sooner than you imagine.

What supplements are right for you?
    <u>A List</u>

    1. multivitamin
    2. antioxidants
    3. tyrosine
    4. meal replacements

    <u>B List</u>

    1. ginkgo, ginseng
    2. caffeine-in moderation (1 cup a day)

5. *Resistance Training* (➤ TOP TEN TOPICS, does lifting weights build muscles in women)

Creative workouts will keep you coming back for more intense workouts. Train with the same kind of passion that you put into your work (hopefully-a lot!!!). Work out with a friend/partner that can motivate you and keep the fire burning.

TRAINING: 3 days a week (Monday, Wednesday, Friday)

A workout right for you!

DAY 1- *MONDAY*

- Circuit train total body
- Perform full circuit 3 times
- No rest between sets within the circuit

- 2 minute rest between circuits
- Males: 8-12 reps, 75-85% failure
- Females: 10-15 reps, 70-80% failure

Circuit #1

1) Bodyweight squats
2) Lat pulldowns
3) Leg curl
4) Calf raises
5) Machine chest press

6) Leg press
7) Standing barbell curls
8) Standing tricep pressdowns
9) 20-30 leg lifts (lying down)
10) Stability ball crunches

REST FOR TWO MINUTES

Circuit #2

Repeat circuit #1 and rest for two minutes.

Circuit #3

Repeat circuit #1/#2.

DAY 2- *WEDNESDAY*

- Power workout
- Lower repetition, longer rest
- 3 sets each exercise
- first set-15 reps to warm up
- MALES: following 2 sets-6-8 reps (85-95% failure)
- WOMEN: following 2 sets-10-12 reps (80-90% failure)

POWER WORKOUT

1) Bench press (flat barbell)
NOTE: Use Smith machine if you don't train w/ a partner
2) Seated lat rows
3) Squats (dumbbells or barbells)
4) Squat thrusts w/ dumbbells
5) Medicine ball crunches
6) Underhand pull ups (use weighted belt if your own bodyweight is not challenging enough)

This workout will certainly give you a run for your money. This is a great outlet for all of your daily stresses or mental restraints. I think that you will accede that this power workout will give you an energy rush that is unparalleled.

HOT NOTE: HIGHER RISK EXERCISES= CAUTION!

❖ ALWAYS train w/ a spotter when it comes to free weight exercises. Otherwise, you could be risking serious debilitating injuries if something slips or is too heavy. Furthermore, if you have any physical limitations (knees, shoulder, lower back pain, etc.), start w/ lighter weights to see how your body reacts to the exercise. TAKE IT SLOW! If you can't perform these exercises, stick to the machines that challenge your muscles.

DAY 3- *FRIDAY*
- Higher repetitions
- 2 sets per body part
- MALES: 15-20 reps, 70-80% failure
- FEMALES: 20-25 reps, 65-75% failure

HOT BODY PARTS
$$$ *Hamstrings, lower back, rear deltoids* $$$

Focus on smaller body parts that may weaken due to being in a prolonged sitting position all day

1) Dumbbell chest press
2) Lying dumbbell tricep extension
3) Lying hamstring curls
4) Rear deltoid raises
5) Dumbbell hammer curls
6) Lat pulldowns
7) Leg extensions
8) Shrugs (dumbbells)
9) Stability ball crunches
10) Low back extensions
11) Side lateral raises

4. *Cardiovascular training*
After you have completed resistance training for the day (Mon/Wed/Fri), perform 15 minutes of interval training and different modes for optimal fat burning.

Monday

Use the x-trainer elliptical for 15 minutes alternating these 2 routines:

	TIME	INTENSITY	HEART RATE
1)	*2 MINUTES*	*SLOW*	*60-65%*
2)	*2 MINUTES*	*FAST*	*80-85%*

Wednesday

Perform a series of step ups and some stepmill work as directed:

TIME	DESCRIPTION
2 MINUTES	*STEP UPS*- alternate legs (on 18 in. box) holding 10 lb. dumbbells (females) or 20 lb. dumbbells (males) in each hand
3 MINUTES	*STEPMILL*- work HR up to 80-85%
1 MINUTE	*STEP UPS*- Just right leg (same weight)
2 MINUTES	*STEPMILL*- HR 80-85%
1 MINUTE	*STEP UPS*- Just left leg (same weight)
2 MINUTES	*STEPMILL*- HR 80-85%
2 MINUTES	*STEP UPS*- Alternate legs (same weight)
2 MINUTES	*STEPMILL*- HR 80-85%
5 MINUTES	*TREADMILL*-cool down walk (if desired)

<u>Friday</u>

"JUMP AROUND" workout!

Note: Carry a watch with you to time your exercises to the best of your ability.

TIME	DESCRIPTION
2 MINUTES	*JUMPING JACKS*
2 MINUTES	*RUNNING*-6.0 mph, 2.0 incline
1 MINUTE	*JUMPING ROPE*
2 MINUTES	*RUNNING*-6.5 mph, 3.0 incline
1 MINUTE	*JUMPING JACKS*
2 MINUTES	*RUNNING*- 7.0 mph, 2.0 incline
1 MINUTE	*JUMPING ROPE*
2 MINUTES	*RUNNING*- 7.0 mph, 3.5 incline
1 MINUTE	*JUMPING JACKS*
1 MINUTE	*RUNNING*- 6.5 mph, 5.0 incline
5 MINUTES	*WALKING*-3.2 mph (cool down)

HOT TIP:
#1

*One day during the week, take a nice 45-minute walk outside alone to clear your mind of any troubles or stresses. Let your mind simply wander. Take in what nature has to offer (hopefully good weather) and appreciate your own existence on this planet. You will come back feeling less tense, refreshed, and ready to go.

3. *Sports*

Enjoy some great outdoor activities either alone or with some friends or relatives (especially on the weekends)
- Rowing/kayaking
- Cross-country/downhill skiing
- Golf (walking)
- Mountain bike riding
- Hiking (for a challenge-attach a 20 lb. backpack)
- Rock climbing* (works all muscle groups)
- Basketball* (moves at varying intensities in game situations)

*All-star selections

2. *How to Move More*　　　　　　　　　　　　　　　　<u>Activity level</u>　　**3.5**

It is all about keeping the body in motion from time to time. Your profession requires less movement during the day than many other professions (ex. builders, electricians, mailmen, policemen, wait staff, etc.). These tips on how to move more will greatly complement the other tips that you have implemented into your daily/weekly schedule.

"Tips to move more for thoughtful thinkers"

- Set a timer of some sort (ex. watch, beeper, computer) to remind you on the hour that it is time to get up and move around. Go outside and get some fresh air if possible.
- Perform 20 body squats every 2 hours.
- Stretch out your hamstrings by touching your toes every few hours.
- Take the stairs wherever possible.
- Drink plenty of water (& you will be forced to get up to use the restroom).
- Have handgrips around.
- Fidget! Move your feet once in a while. This will burn an additional 150 calories a day!

1. *Obstacles and Ways To Conquer Them* (❧ all TOP TEN TOOLS)

1. Stress	Stay focused on your health first! Do not become consumed in your work and neglect your health. Your work will subsequently falter if you don't pay mind to your well being. Cook your all-star foods & train consistently. This will do wonders for your stress level and your energy level. You will have that youthful appearance and feel rejuvenated once again!
2. Sitting and using your brilliantly creative mind for long periods of time	Follow the prescribed tips for "moving more". Sit with good posture. This will keep everything flowing and allow for a consistent flow of energy throughout your entire body. Overall, you will have more energy, clarity, alertness, and readiness to create a brilliant idea!
3. Spending time alone	Post up positive sayings in your work environment. Listen to positive, uplifting music. Feed your mind with positive info from various books. Call up a friend once in a while just to talk or maybe even workout with him. Leave work at work. Enjoy time away w/ family & friends. Don't be afraid to interact competitively; engage in various sports/activities mentioned.

	Activity Level	Stress Level
	5.5	8.0

15. SALES & MARKETING ☎

It's part of the job!

You are highly energetic ready to pitch a great offer! You deal with people on a daily basis (sometimes for long hours). Schmoozing, wining & dining your potential clients are all part of the business. You may be on the road traveling in different areas day-to-day, meeting prospective clients.

You are highly motivated and self-disciplined. You are goal-oriented in what you do and despite hearing the word "NO" (dealing with negative reinforcement), you remain positive in the face of naysayers. Your creativity, innovation, & selling strategies are well tuned and constantly being refined for bigger and better sells. The attitude & personality that you bring to the table is what drives your successes. You are highly charismatic & successful at what you do, not letting the fear of failure stop you from achieving your goals. You embrace challenges like a champion!

10. *Lifestyle Tips*

Carry your internal drive to achieve success at your job into the gym and with your eating habits. You will have no problem achieving great successes in your overall health and wellness when you transport your high-octane nature & great work ethic with you into your workouts and diet. Stay proactive and get on a fitness program that works especially for you with your schedule, and stay consistent. Hold yourself accountable by seeing a physical trainer each week to chart your progress.

When meeting a client at a restaurant, be disciplined in the type of food that you choose to eat and in your alcohol intake. You will make a statement that exudes confidence and value in yourself. Your potential customers will be impressed with how much professionalism you display and will be more apt to believe and follow what you say.

When you are traveling from place to place, it is very important to be stocked with energizing, healthy foods. Even when you are not traveling and you are at your desk or specific location, bring these "all-star" foods with you. This will make a world of difference for your mentality when dealing with people.

At various times, your stress level may be through the roof if a big sale is in the works. Whether it is cars, furniture, high-tech software, on-line goods, properties, you name it, your yearly salary is based largely on how much you sell. As you well know, there are those slump periods where you hear "no" for many different reasons. Don't get too low, take the good with the bad and have a healthy outlet like exercise or a favorite sport to enjoy. Remember, your health is first and foremost in importance. Money can be made back at any age; your health is precious at every age of your life, so take care of it!

9. All-Star Foods and Liquid Fuel (☎ TOP TEN FIT FAST FOODS)

FOODS/LIQUID FUEL TO BRING ON THE ROAD

➤ Caffeine & alcohol in moderation (1 cup/glass every other day)
➤ Green tea (contains antioxidants-excellent for a stressful profession)
➤ Water (120 oz.)
➤ Most grocery stores have an array of healthy, inexpensive foods choices (fruits/veggies/salad bars)
➤ Dining at restaurants-grilled foods, sushi, salad bar, mixed veggies (limit carbohydrates consumed, avoid airplane/airport foods)

SNACKS ON THE ROAD

Clif bars	protein bars	Brazil nuts
meal replacements	Kashi Go-Lean bars	sunflower seeds
Grapenuts	almonds	apples
Breathsavers/sugarless gum	pumpkin seeds	peanut butter on rye

FOODS FOR THE OFFICE

➤ Turkey breast (4 oz.) on pumpernickel, deli pickle, cucumber salad
➤ Grilled chicken breast, sweet potato, carrot sticks
➤ Low-fat yogurt, cottage cheese, lite mozzarella sticks, soymilk, tofu
➤ Chicken soup, flaxseed chips, wheat pitas
➤ Pears, prunes, raisins, mangos, oranges

FOODS AT HOME

➤ Egg whites, oatmeal, orange juice
➤ Large tossed salad w/ grilled chicken breast strips, celery, olive oil & vinegar, tomatoes
➤ Roasted turkey breast, chili, barley
➤ Lean meat (top round sirloin steak), flank steak, baked potato, mixed steamed veggies
➤ Salmon, swordfish, halibut, shrimp, brown rice, asparagus

8. Foods to Avoid (☎ TOP TEN TOPICS, alcohol)

➤ **Caffeine:** Limit your intake. Your energy levels are naturally high so additional stimulants are not necessary. (ex. café mochas, café lattes, light & sweet flavored coffee)

➢ **Alcohol:** You will dehydrate yourself with too much. Empty, low-nutritive value drinks simply mean wasteful calories added. Excessive amounts are physically detrimental over a period of time.

➢ **High-fat fast foods:** We are faced with temptations and the lack of control our society has (as a whole) for eating these high-calorie, high-fat food items. Many fast food restaurants are introducing many low-fat, healthier items to their menu.

➢ **Gas station snacks:** donuts, burritos, buttered popcorn, granola bars, candy, cookies, soda, slushies, hot dogs

➢ **Big dinners:** In today's society, many restaurants are serving larger portions. For example, a typical pasta dinner in America will contain 6-7 servings of pasta vs. a typical pasta dinner in Italy (2-3 servings).

➢ **High cheese foods:** pizza, macaroni & cheese, nachos, chicken parmigiana, eggplant parmigiana

7. *Meals: How many & when?*

If it is a "non-workout" day, eat small, frequent moderate carb/high protein meals every 3 hours. As the night progresses, reduce your carb intake & up your protein levels. Do not eat past 8 P.M. (as a general rule).

*Schedule for meals on your workout days:

BIG BREAKFAST	7 A.M.
SMALL SNACK	10 A.M.
WORKOUT	12 P.M.
MEAL REPLACEMENT	1 P.M.
MEDIUM-SIZED MEAL	2 P.M.
SMALL MEAL	5 P.M.
SMALL MEAL	7:30 P.M.

*Your schedule may vary from this. Use same intervals relative to your individual schedule.

6. *Supplementation & Sleep*

Clear your mind of all of the day's highs & lows. You have worked hard to make that sale, trained hard to better your wellness, and now it is time to REST like a champion! It shouldn't be a problem getting a minimum of 7 hours of sleep a night. The harder you have worked, the better you will sleep. If you don't get the proper rest necessary, over time your focus at work will falter. You won't feel like training and only your wallet will appear a bit thinner.

What supplements are right for you?

    <u>A List</u>

    1. multivitamin
    2. antioxidant
    3. vitamin B (100 mg)
    4. glutamine
    5. tyrosine
    6. meal replacements

    <u>B List</u>

    1. ZMA
    2. melatonin

5. *Resistance Training* (☎ TOP TEN TOPICS, is spot reducing possible)

Working out mid-day would suit you best. This will give you something to look forward to during the morning time and make the day fly by thereafter. Additionally, this will kick start your energy for the remainder of the day. Your performance will be that much better for later on when many of your potential clients are available.

A workout right for you!

- Monday/Thursday= UPPER BODY
- Tuesday/Friday= LOWER BODY

<u>MONDAY</u>

❑ **One minute rest between sets**
    1) 100 pushups (4 sets of 25 reps w/ varying grips)
        • shoulder-width (sets 1 & 3)-hands even w/ mid-pec region
        • diamond pushups(sets 2 &4)- make a diamond out of your hands connecting your index fingers and thumbs and keep your hands directly below your chest
    2) 50 pull ups (5 sets of 10 reps w/ varying grips)
        • shoulder-width overhand
        • shoulder-width underhand
        • wide grip (approx. 2 inches wider than shoulder-width)
        • narrow grip (approx. 2 inches closer than shoulder-width)
        • shoulder-width overhand

NOTE: Use assisted pull up machine if you can't do the pull ups on your own.
   3) 50 dips (2 sets-25 reps/set)
   4) 20 bicep curls (2 sets-20 reps/set-85% failure on last 2 reps)

TUESDAY

- ☐ superset lower body workout (do each superset 3 times)
- ☐ 1 minute rest between supersets
- ☐ no rest between exercises within the superset
- ☐ **FEMALES: 15 reps, 80-85% failure on last 2 reps**
  MALES: 10 reps, 85-90% failure on last 2 reps

SUPERSET 1:

1) Squats	1) Squats	1) Squats
2) Leg extensions	2) Leg extensions	2) Leg extensions
rest for 1 minute	rest for 1 minute	rest for 1 minute, on to superset 2

SUPERSET 2:

Repeat same format above for:

   1) Lying leg curl
   2) Seated leg curl

SUPERSET 3:

Repeat same format above for:

   1) Standing calf raises
   2) Seated calf raises

SUPERSET 4: (CORE TRI-SET)

Repeat same format above for the following **3 exercises at 15 reps/exercise**

   1) Stability ball crunches

2) Hanging leg raises
3) Supermans

THURSDAY

❑   superset upper body workout (do each superset 3 times)
❑   1 minute rest between supersets
❑   no rest between exercises within the supersets
❑   **FEMALES: 15 reps, 80-90% failure on last 2 reps**
    MALES: 10 reps, 85-95% failure on last 2 reps

SUPERSET 1:

1) Lat pulldown   1) Lat pulldown   1) Lat pulldown
2) Standing barbell   2) Standing barbell   2) Standing barbell

rest for 1 minute   rest for 1 minute   rest for 1 minute,
                                              on to superset 2

SUPERSET 2:

Repeat same format above for:

5) Dumbbell bench press
6) Lying dumbbell tricep extensions

SUPERSET 3:

Repeat same format above for:

1) Seated lat row
2) Seated dumbbell shoulder press

SUPERSET 4:

Repeat same format above for:

1) Incline chest press
2) Side lateral raises

FRIDAY

- ❑ **One minute rest between sets**
- ❑ **For a "shredded" lower body**

1) 30-50 body weight squats*
2) 1 min- walking lunges
3) 2 min-step ups on 18-inch bench holding 10 lb. dumbbells in each arm
4) 20 lying leg curls (3 sets-80% failure on last 2 reps/set)
5) 2 min-jumping jacks
6) 20 standing calf raises (3 sets-80% failure on last 2 reps/set)
7) 1 min-wall squat
8) 25 body weight squats*

*Gauge your own fitness levels accordingly.

HOT TIP:

#1

*Compete with yourself each time that you go the gym. Make up a game with yourself where you set up goals to achieve in the gym and the higher levels you obtain there, the more sales you will make, also. You will be surprised at how one facet of your life can positively translate into another.

4. Cardiovascular training

- ❑ **3 days a week (Mon/Tue/Thur) for 15 minutes**
- ❑ **Perform intervals & use a different mode each day:**

Use the x-trainer, treadmill, & stepmill (each on different days), following this interval schedule for each day:

TIME	INTERVAL	HEART RATE
3 min	slow & easy	60-70%
2 min	fast & hard	80-85%

REPEAT THIS 3 TIMES (for a total of 15 minutes)

3. *Sports*

You enjoy the thrill of victory when it arrives! A good quality of a good salesman/marketing genius is being very competitive & passionate in what he/she is offering. You are always setting the standard and trying to raise the bar for yourself (& possibly others).

Engage in some competitive sports in which you will excel.

- Flag football leagues
- Rec basketball leagues
- Road races
- Bowling leagues
- Softball leagues
- Golf leagues

2. *How to Move More*   <u>Activity level</u>   <u>5.5</u>

If you are one that travels frequently, sit with good posture. Focus on your sales pitch or presentation. Remember to bring your water with you and drink it consistently. Every hour, you should need to stop and use the restroom. Do 15 squats while you are out of the car and stretch by touching your toes and holding for 15 seconds and then touching for the sky and holding for another 15 seconds. Walk, talk, and move with confidence & good posture. A positive, believable attitude sells!

You are energetic & charismatic by nature (whether you feel like that at any given time is another story), but you are the consummate professional. You are always on and must be channeled in to sweep people off their feet with a great "win-win" proposition. In order to be in the zone, you must keep up your metabolic rate through physical activity and eating well throughout the day.

If you are working indoors and usually sitting all day, get up on the hour and do 10 body squats. Walk around in the office and stay busy. If you can't get up for long time frames, then fidget at your seat to keep your body active.

1. *Obstacles and Ways To Conquer Them*

1. Being on your game at all times	Train hard & challenge yourself outside of work. You will gain a sense of accomplishment & self-confidence and know that if you can sell yourself to this concept of SUPER HEALTH, then you can achieve anything (with a plan, of course). Eat your all-star foods regularly and no matter what happens at work (good or bad), smile at least 30 times a day. It is much easier to smile than frown!

2. Finding time to workout

Keep a slot open for exercise on a regular basis. Just as you would find time to meet a potential customer for a sale, you should find time to train hard and make a SUPER HEALTH profit that is immeasurable & priceless. There is no reason ever to sacrifice your well being!

3. Resting appropriately and avoiding burnout with a high-stress level

Take time for yourself and participate in activities that you enjoy. Life is about taking the good with the bad and staying confident in yourself, throughout. Continue to take an interest in people and help someone else with a need. This will take the focus off yourself & allow you to make another type of impact to benefit society.

4. Traveling & working long hours

Refer to the section on "Moving More". You can increase your metabolic rate at work with the tips that we provide. Continue to eat your all-star foods regularly & once a month you can go all out and indulge in your favorite dishes. The battle is half won at this point. If you are on the road frequently, make it a priority to find a gym immediately. Think about this,4 out of 112 awake available hours during the week is not too much time devoted for an investment into your SUPER HEALTH account! You will live the multi-million dollar lifestyle already by following your customized plan for overall wellness.

	Activity Level	Stress Level
	7.0	4.5

16. SERVICE INDUSTRY ✂

It's part of the job!

You are what you do! Your actions speak louder than your words. You are always giving of your time and energy to help others. You are always selling yourself and your abilities on a daily basis. Therefore, you need to present a good image to others so that they not only hear what you preach, but believe in it. Being a picture of good health is very important in your profession.

You are very hands-on and practical in your approaches with people. In many ways, you represent an industry of your product so the pressure is on to perform, as you would tell others to perform. For example, as a personal trainer, you would advise your clients to eat certain foods and lift weights using certain techniques and strategies that hopefully you, too, would implement in your own lifestyle. Your activity level is high throughout the day so you want to eat, train, and rest right so your tank remains full while you are at work.

10. *Lifestyle Tips*

Take care of yourself FIRST. Believe it or not, you are a role model for your clients. If you can't take care of yourself, your words will not carry much weight and you won't be able to provide adequate service for your people. Find activities that you really enjoy and take the time to engage in them. Balance your workload with leisure activities.

You must be very competent at your profession for people to listen to your words. Having accreditations, certifications, and proper education is a prerequisite for properly instructing others on how to excel in that specific field or simply providing a fair, just service to others.

Stick to the principles that you preach. Being in a business for a long period of time could cause one to get complacent, even hypocritical to his/her own philosophies. Telling others what they need to do in order to better themselves and achieve their personal goals is good. But, when you begin to slip, yourself, and stop honing your own skills or simply stop taking care of yourself, then your cliental will become aware. Keep the expectations for yourself and others high. Continue to raise the bar for your own standards!

Your activity level is high throughout the day, so make sure that you bring your all-star foods to work and monitor how active you are. Proper rest is essential for effectiveness at work. Workouts will greatly benefit your physical and mental wellness. You can vary your workouts making them fun and different. We show you some ways to do that.

9. All-Star Foods and Liquid Fuel

FOODS AT WORK

a. Pure protein bars, meal replacements, Luna bars, Clif bars

b. Low-fat yogurt, cottage cheese, hard-boiled eggs, Brazil nuts, sunflower seeds

c. Tuna fish (albacore) on rye bread, sweet potato/yam, pickle

d. Grilled chicken breast, leafy green salads (w/ olive oil, tomatoes, olives, celery, spinach, cucumbers)-low calorie, high-fiber veggies

HOT TIP:
#1

*Check out the "Top 10 Fit-Fast Foods" if you want to switch it up or take a client out to eat.

FOODS AT HOME

1) Grilled eggplant w/ olive oil, 8 oz. of turkey breast, pumpernickel bread

2) Oatmeal (old-fashioned, non-instant), 3 egg whites, 1 egg yolk, orange juice/grape juice

3) Asparagus, beans (all kinds), lean pork tenderloin

4) Fish (salmon, swordfish, shrimp), brown rice, sliced mushroom & zucchini

5) Top round & sirloin cuts of meat, grilled veggies, baked potato w/ hot sauce

Liquid Fuel

¾ **gallon water**-bring a gallon and you will be able to gauge how much to drink daily

8. Foods to Avoid (✂ TOP TEN TOPICS, glycemic index)

High sugar (high GI) foods that pick you up quickly will also drop your energy levels quickly. With your energy levels being high, you need to fuel your body with long-lasting energy (low GI foods).

A) <u>High GI foods</u>

Examples:

     donuts   French bread

     bagels   cookie dough ice cream

     mashed potatoes   pretzels

     vanilla wafers

B) <u>Caffeinated beverages</u>

NOTE: Avoid getting addicted to coffee and other caffeinated beverages. Caffeine is an anti-nutrient and limits your calcium availability in bones & muscles in the body.

AVOID: lattes, mochas, light & sweet flavored coffees

C) <u>Frequent dining out at restaurants</u>

D) <u>Frozen entrees, processed foods</u>

E) <u>Creamy dressings on salads</u>

F) <u>Trans-fat products</u>

Examples: **margarine, fried foods, bacon**

7. *Meals: How many & when?*

Five to six small meals a day eaten every 3 hours will consistently supply nutrients throughout your body providing a stable amount of energy throughout the day. This will keep your body on a 24-hour a day fat burning marathon. This method of eating will promote muscle growth without gaining excess fat storage.

Get yourself into this eating schedule using the all-star food choices that we recommend for 6 days a week. Then, for one day a week, you can eat whatever your heart desires.

*Consume a meal replacement directly following a workout session.

6. Supplementation & Sleep

Eight hours of rest consistently is a must. Your schedule may be at odd hours based on your clients' availability. Do not schedule late evenings and early mornings back to back. To avoid becoming a "burnout casualty", plan your scheduling so you can get the consistent 8 hours of sleep a night.

What supplements are right for you?

<u>A</u> List

1. multivitamin (2 a day-1 in morning, 1 at lunch-due to high activity)
2. creatine/glutamine (males)-1 month on, 2 weeks off (5 grams-morning, 5 grams-post-training)
3. caffeine, 200 mgs right before training
4. antioxidant

<u>B</u> List

1. NO2 (males)
2. tyrosine, ginkgo, ginseng
3. ZMA

5. Resistance Training

Whether you are a hairdresser, trainer, massage therapist, coach, martial arts, aerobics, voice, or dance instructor, you want your students/cliental to feel their best. You earn a living by challenging them and making sure that you show them how to get stronger, more agile, or just look and feel better in the area that you specialize in.

Incorporating different movements into your own workouts is something that you may be able to utilize with your clients or classes. Having this knowledge will definitely add to your prowess as being "the expert" and role model. Your ultimate goal can be to become an all-around expert, the jack-of all trades.

NOTE: Before you proceed forward, the following workout is for the very conditioned. This workout will keep your body in tremendous tip-top shape. If you don't think that you are quite ready for something of this magnitude, refer to the "Top 10 Topics" and try "The best workout you've never done" for 3 months. Then, come back and try this workout. Anyone can obtain great results from this workout.

A workout right for you!

DAY 1- *MONDAY*

- Upper body
- Stability workout

- Will recruit many muscle groups not normally used
- MALES: 3 sets, 8-10 reps, 75-85% failure on last 2 reps
- FEMALES: 3 sets, 10-15 reps, 75-85% failure on last 2 reps

1. DUMBBELL BENCH PRESS

    o   Lying on a stability ball (pretend the ball is a bench), rest your shoulders and head on ball. Knees and feet should be off the ball, but stable.

2. STANDING BICEP CURLS

    o   Hold dumbbells and tubing in both hands. Wrap the tubing under your feet. This is very challenging and creates constant resistance.

3. SIDE RAISES (standing on left foot)

4. DUMBBELL SHOULDER PRESSES (standing on right foot)

5. PULLUPS (hold a medicine ball between your knees)

6. ONE ARM CABLE ROWS (standing on opposite foot)

    o   Right arm rowing=standing on left foot (and vice versa)
        Line up cable in the middle of your stomach.

7. 30 PUSHUPS (feet on stability ball, hands on the ground)

DAY 2- *TUESDAY*

THE "ONE LEG" WORKOUTS

Same repetition scheme as Monday

1)   25 squats to warm up
2)   1 leg-leg extensions (right foot-1st, left foot-2nd for all exercises)
3)   1 leg-leg curls (seated)
4)   1 leg-step ups holding dumbbells stepping onto an 18-in. box or bench
5)   1 leg calf raises standing

6)   stability ball crunches
7)   hanging leg raises holding stability ball between knees

DAY 3- *THURSDAY*

PLYOMETRIC POWER WORKOUT

a.   2 SETS- 25 hand-clap pushups
b.   2 SETS- 25 box jumps (find an 18-24 inch stable platform, jump on it, then jump back on ground, then immediately back on the box)
c.   2 SETS- 10 pull ups (vary grips-underhand, overhand)
     (use assisted machine if you can't perform a regular pull up)
d.   2 SETS- 25 jump squats
e.   2 SETS- 20 lateral hops (set up a 12x12 inch box, hop over it side to side laterally 20 times)
f.   2 MINUTES-jump rope
g.   2 SETS-20 abdominal crunches w/ medicine ball held directly over head

DAY 4- *SATURDAY*

HEAD-TO-TOE CIRCUIT

- Through all 3 circuits
- 2 minute rest between circuits
- no rest between exercises within the circuit
- HR 60% maintained
- MALES: 10 reps
- FEMALES: 12 reps

Circuit #1

1. Machine chest press
2. Lat row
3. Seated preacher curls
4. Standing tricep extensions
5. Machine shoulder press
6. Leg press
7. Lying leg curl
8. Low back extensions
9. Jumping jacks

REST FOR 2 MINUTES

<u>Circuit #2</u>

1-8-same as circuit #1
9. 2 minutes- jump rope

REST FOR 2 MINUTES

<u>Circuit #3</u>

1-8-same as circuits #1,#2
9. 2 minutes-walking lunges

4. *Cardiovascular training*
After you have completed resistance training for the day (Mon/Tue/Thur), perform 15-20 minutes of aerobic workouts at varying intensities.

<u>Monday</u>

INTENSE WIND SPRINTS AT THE TRACK

- 100 yard dash, walk back to start
- 50 yard dash, walk back to start
- repeat this sequence 5 times for a total of 10 sprints

<u>Tuesday</u>

HILLSPRINTS

- find a good sized hill (100-150 ft.)
- 60% grade would be ideal
- sprint up the hill, walk back down
- repeat 10 times

<u>Thursday</u>

JOG 2 MILES

3. *Sports*

Many of you pride yourselves on your daily appearance. If you have a good athletic background, why not continue to challenge yourself in these different forms of advanced competitions. Even if you aren't into many sports, trying new activities can not hurt.

Enjoy some competitive activities sure to get your juices flowing:
- bodybuilding
- triathlons
- biathlons
- marathons
- cross-country skiing

2. *How to Move More*   Activity level   7.0

If you are actively implementing your customized resistance training program along with your cardio-vascular program and giving all of your mental, physical, and emotional energy to your clients/customers, then you will not need any tips for moving more. Just remember to feed yourself the all-star selections recommended. The only tip that we have for you is to find more time to relax and cherish your time off. Stand tall (chest up, abs tight, head & shoulders back) and look strong. You are a model of what you preach and what you do!

1. *Obstacles and Ways To Conquer Them* (✂ all TOP TEN RESULTS)

1. Staying motivated on a consistent basis	We sound like a broken record, but the truth is that your cliental relies heavily on your overall wellness. Be aware of that and give 110% to yourself and it won't be a problem giving it to your clients, also. Stay disciplined!
2. Burning out	Monitor how long and hard you are working. We know that hard work pays off, but realize that you should enjoy your time off and relax a bit. It will do your body wonders. Refer to your tips on sleep.
3. Standing on your feet all day	Many of you are on your feet all day. The pull of gravity down on your feet can take a toll on your entire body. Stand tall and purchase a comfortable pair of shoes. You will be using them over 1/3 of the day.

Activity Level	Stress Level
9.5	3.0

17. SKILLED MANUAL LABORERS 🛠

It's part of the job! (🛠 TOP TEN TOPICS, proper form)

Your job is very demanding on your body. You are always working with your hands and are on your feet. Your muscles require an extremely high amount of sustained energy. Moving, lifting, climbing, twisting, fixing, screwing, unscrewing, squatting, reaching, bending, you name it, describe what, often times, you do on a daily basis.

A problem area for many of you is your back. You have to be very careful not to throw your back out or develop serious problems with postural alignment over the years. Your back can support a great amount of weight and often times we are unaware of how much undue stress our back takes for our entire body. We provide techniques for you to use to help strengthen your back, assisting in preventing any (further) complications.

Often times, your schedule represents long hours during good weather days and limited work, at times, when the weather is bad. Many times, lots of beer and junk food coincide with one another during those long days. Negative co-workers may influence your attitude at work. We show you how a little discipline can go a long way towards achieving SUPER HEALTH.

10. *Lifestyle Tips*

You would think that the physical labor that you do on a daily basis would be enough for exercise & fitness. Your body adapts to every physical situation that it encounters. The type of fuel that you put into your body matters greatly! The theory that garbage in equals garbage out holds true. If you consistently fuel your body with food products such as beer, loaded high fat meat grinders (sausage, meatball), sloppy joes, and chips, then your body will have no choice but to operate as instructed by its type of fuel. Your body will go through great energy swings many times resulting in a lethargic state of mind and body.

When you perform your workouts in the gym, keep them short & intense. Spend a great deal of focus on strengthening your back (especially lower back) and legs.

Feed the machine regularly! Refrain from eating 2 big meals during the day. Let's face it, you are a hard worker. Therefore, instead of developing poor eating habits, let your body experience high quality proteins and low GI carbohydrates on a frequent basis (every 3-4 hours). Your body will adapt in a positive way to format itself ready for muscle toning. As a result, this will help you excel in the trade that you are proficient.

9. All-Star Foods and Liquid Fuel

FOODS FROM HOME

➢ Whole wheat pasta, ground turkey breast, & carrot sticks
➢ Grilled chicken breast, brown rice, sauteed broccoli, & red pepper (in olive oil)
➢ Sliced turkey breast on wheat pita
➢ Leafy green salads w/ olive oil & vinegar (spinach, olives, carrots, cucumbers, tomatoes-contain lycopene-a potent antioxidant)

SNACKS AT WORK

➢ Apples (aids digestion of fatty foods)
➢ Pears
➢ Peaches
➢ Strawberries
➢ Pure protein bars
➢ Meal replacements

HOT TIP:
#1

*Carry your meal replacements with you. Whether they are in your lunch bag, work bag, or vehicle, having nutritional bars or a shaker container to mix up approximately 40 grams of high-quality protein is of the utmost importance to keep those muscles that you use all day consistently fueled.

ON-THE-ROAD FOODS

➢ Subway grinders (whole wheat bread w/ lean cuts of meat-turkey, chicken, tuna fish w/ veggies, hot sauce, hot peppers, no cheese or mayo needed)
➢ Oatmeal (old-fashioned, non-instant) in morning (2 cups) w/ honey, 1% milk, Splenda, & grape juice, low-fat yogurt (starting out the morning strong will give you an unbelievable reserve of energy throughout the day)
➢ Eggs (yolks contain biotin-growth factor from B-complex vitamins)

NOTE: Intense training & work cause a buildup of lactic acid in muscles. Biotin is an integral part of helping to break down lactic acid buildup.
➢ Consume 1-2 whole eggs a day, have 3-4 egg whites (preferably at breakfast). You could mix up this 4-6 egg combo in an omelette w/ olive oil, spinach, & peppers.
➢ Sunflower seeds, sesame seeds, almonds, Brazil nuts

➢   Sweet potatoes (high in beta-carotene), yams, red potatoes, cottage cheese
➢   Fish (salmon, halibut, swordfish) & barley bean soup
➢   Lean red meat (flank, top round sirloin, 90% fat-free ground beef-contains essential amino acids)-helps create an anabolic (muscle-building) environment in your body

Liquid Fuel

•   Consume 1 gallon of water daily, especially if you work outdoors in the hot sun. You must stay hydrated.

8. *Foods to Avoid*

Your buddies at work may often splurge and probably enjoy many of these All-American meals at any time of the day. You are a high riser and will obtain a state of SUPER HEALTH if you pay careful attention to avoid the following foods.

➢   Pizza and beer
➢   Sausage & pepper grinders, sloppy joes, meatball & cheese grinders on white bread/grinder rolls
➢   Donuts, muffins, light & sweet flavored coffees
NOTE: Drinking caffeinated beverages on a regular basis will set your hard-working body up for bouts of dehydration and fatigue.
➢   Quick hit snacks: chips, nachos, cookies, soda, ice cream
➢   Pastrami, salami, bologna, pepperoni, roast beef cold cuts
➢   Whole milk cheeses (cheddar, Swiss, jack), whole milk
➢   Pancakes w/ maple syrup, frozen waffles w/ strawberry topping & whipped cream
➢   Processed dinner aids

7. *Meals: How many & when?*

The biggest obstacle for many of you is eating at the correct times. Many times, you get involved with your work and you need to be here one minute and over there, the next. Often times, you get into your work routine and end up consuming a large lunch and an even larger dinner late at night. This is due to the fact that you have expended much of your energy during the day and your body requires a refueling (that is if you didn't follow our tips and bring your all-star food choices with you to work).

Having a big dinner w/ some alcohol is not the late night answer. Why? Gauge your activity level at night compared to the daytime. Your activity level is low, if not active at all in the hours after you get home from work. You may just want to sit down and sit in front of the tube, pop a few brews and enjoy a baseball game after a long, exhausting day at work. When your food intake is high while your metabolism decreases and your activity level is low, your body begins to store calories in the most inopportune places. The solution that we provide takes a bit of consistency and good habit formation and at first it is a bit of a challenge to acquire. Like anything else, once you get started, your body will adapt and respond like a champion. Put these tools in your tool belt everyday, set them in motion, and you will discover untapped potential.

- EAT A SOUND, NUTRITIOUS BREAKFAST IMMEDIATELY UPON WAKING UP
  This should be your "biggest" meal of the day. Choose from the all-star food selections and provide your body with energy that will allow you to function at an optimal level throughout the day. This will prevent your muscles from breaking down in search of needed energy that has been lost throughout the day. An added bonus is that you will have the energy to hit the gym after work!

- BRING MEAL REPLACEMENTS WITH YOU TO WORK
  Consume meal replacements on a frequent basis (every 2-3 hours). This will add 40 grams of quality protein that your body needs. Instead of a coffee and cigarette break, try our "PROTEIN-POWER" break. It's very easy to mix in a shaker w/ some ice water out of your gallon.

- EAT A MEDIUM-SIZED LUNCH AND DINNER
  Again, choose from the all-star food choices list for a lunch that will keep you going. If you have taken in your other foods correctly up until now, the rest of the ride home will be that much easier until your head hits the pillow.

Here's the breakdown:

6 A.M.	Largest meal-breakfast
9 A.M.	meal replacement (protein power break)
12 P.M.	medium-sized lunch
3 P.M.	protein power break/all-star snack break
5 P.M.	protein power break/all-star snack break
7:30 P.M.	small-med-sized dinner (low carb)

6. Supplementation & Sleep

Your profession is one of the highest rated for 8 hours of sleep, bar none!

What supplements are right for you?

A List

1. multivitamin (1-morning & 1-night)-due to increased daily energy expenditure
2. creatine/glutamine (5 grams-morning, 5 grams-post-training)-4 weeks on, one week off=better strength & recovery

3. antioxidants- help fight free radicals, which are a byproduct of intense exercise (high in vitamin C & E)

4. vitamin B (100 mg)

<u>B List</u>

1. ZMA

2. HMB

3. glucosamine/chondroitin

4. caffeine (pre-training-200 mg, 1 medium cup of black coffee)

5. *Resistance Training* (✕ TOP TEN TOPICS, the best workout you have never done)

Two words: SHORT, INTENSE

Four days: 3 days during week, 1 day on weekend

Duration: 30 minutes

Type of training: HIGH-INTENSE STRENGTH TRAINING

(4 day-split body parts)

➤ During the week, train at the same time every day after work.

➤ An hour after you have completed work for the day is the best time for training.

➤ Consume a meal replacement right after work.

➤ 200 mg. caffeine before training will give you that kickstart to your workout.

A workout right for you!

- FEMALES: 3 sets/exercise, 10-12 reps, 85-95% failure on last 2-3 reps
- MALES: 3 sets/exercise, 6-8 reps; 90-99% failure on last 2-3 reps

<u>DAY 1</u> **Chest, Triceps**

1) Bench press (barbells)

2) Lying tricep extensions (2 dumbbells)

3) Incline dumbbell press (20 degree incline)

4) Standing tricep pressdowns

5) Machine crunches for abs

<u>DAY 2</u> **Back, Biceps**

1) Seated lat row

2) Standing barbell curls

3) Lat pulldowns
4) Seated hammer curl dumbbells
5) Low back extensions, 45 deg. bench-hold weight on your chest

DAY 3 Legs

1) Squats (barbells)
2) Stiff leg deadlifts, slight bend in knees
3) Standing calf raises
4) Leg extensions
5) Hanging leg raises holding medium ball between ankles

DAY 4 Shoulders

1) Dumbbell seated shoulder press
2) Barbell shrugs
3) Side lateral raises
4) Rear delt flyes
5) Internal & external rotations (light weight, no failure, 1set of 25 reps both ways)

HOT BODY PARTS
$$$ LOW BACK $$$

Along with the exercise that you do for your back on "back day", make low back extensions a mainstay in your training. We are thinking for the long haul for you to maintain/increase strength, flexibility, and posture.

Before you go to bed, every other night perform 15 supermans by raising your legs and arms up at the same time holding that position for 2 seconds.

$$$ SHOULDERS$$$

Warm up these small muscle groups prior to training any part of your upper body. 50 small arm circles to the front and rear performed along with your internal and external rotations on your shoulder day will do the trick.

$$$ LEGS $$$

Try and execute 15 squats each day either in the morning, lunch or nighttime.

4. *Cardiovascular training*

Your workweek is intense enough! Adding further rigorous cardio to your week will be counterproductive resulting in inevitable burnout and muscle catabolism. Work hard at your job and eat correctly and you will be good to go!

Once on the weekend, walk or cycle on the stationary bike for 30-45 minutes low & slow maintaining a heart rate at 60-70% (best in morning).

If your workweek gets reduced due to inclement weather, then after your resistance training (3 out of the 4 days), you can engage in cardio training for 20 minutes at the same low/slow intensity (60-70% HR).

3. *Sports*
Enjoy some relaxing, yet friendly competitive sports.

- Softball league
- Golfing league
- Yoga & Pilates-gets the body in proper alignment and keeps muscles long and supple

2. *How to Move More*   <u>Activity level</u>   <u>9.5</u>

Your activity level throughout the day tells the story. You guys (& girls) are extremely active working your tails off, constantly moving and working strenuously.

Here is the catch, when you are "moving more", always be aware of your body. Throughout the day, you will be working in many different situations placing your body in awkward positions. On top of that, many of you will be wearing a tool belt so be conscious and never let your low back be placed in a compromising position. Use those strong legs that you have built up for support rather than adding strain to your lower back. When you have to work in those varying positions, do it with good posture. Draw in your navel into your spine. This will prevent against any abdominal distention, which may result in lower back pain.

From time to time throughout the day, you can stretch those hamstrings of yours out by bending over at the waist and touching your toes holding the stretch for 10 seconds.

1. *Obstacles and Ways To Conquer Them*

| 1. Lack of energy at the end of the day to workout | Be disciplined on a daily basis with your meal replacements, big breakfast & small meals frequently. Stick with it and stay consistent. Get your required 8 hours of beauty sleep. If you need to take a 10 min. nap after work prior to working out, do so. Take the 100-200 mg of caffeine pre-training to rev up the engine. |

2. Weaker, overworked back and body

Watch developing the infamous "beer belly". This is one of the primary causes of lower back pain and a compromised lower back. Perform your low back exercises every other night. Watch your posture. Develop good habits!

3. Eating well around a negative-eating environment

You are a high-riser and do not want to settle for just mediocrity. You realize that eating well is 80% of the overall journey towards SUPER HEALTH achievement.

Activity Level	Stress Level
5.5	5.5

18. STAY AT HOME MOTHERS ♀

It's part of the job!

This may be the most challenging and the most important of all professional fields that we cover. Don't let anyone tell you otherwise; being a full-time mom is a full-time job and is absolutely invaluable! Your child requires your undivided attention throughout the day. Often times, there are those sleepless nights where any distraction heard may be something you need to attend to. You are more than just a mother figure to your child. You are a role model! You set the example early on in your child's life for many of their habits including eating habits and lifestyle habits. On top of that, if you are a new mother, in the process of tending to your child's daily needs, you may be wondering how you can go back to that pre-pregnancy appearance/weight and shed off the added pounds that can accompany a pregnancy. We understand that there is a lot on your plate here, certainly more than meets the eye.

10. *Lifestyle Tips*

Habits form early on in life and it is up to you to start your children off on firm ground and teach them proper dietary habits and the type of lifestyle that will benefit them throughout their lives. You can be the most powerful teacher of all by demonstrating through example just what you want them to establish for habits. Actions speak louder than words!!

Choose to live right by eating well. You have the power to choose what it is that your children do and do not eat. Choose wisely for them and they will reap the rewards as they get older. Also, engage in active, fun activities for many reasons. Children need to move and release any pent up stored energy. Their minds require a stimulation that exercise provides. Try to limit their amount of time in front of the television set and sitting around doing other sedentary activities.

Getting back to your personal routine, you could find time to work out early in the morning while your husband and child are still sleeping or before your husband goes to work. This early morning workout will elevate your energy levels throughout the entire day, which is often times what you lack with such a demanding responsibility. Get your husband on board and tell him how important it is for you to get into tip-top shape. Any good husband would be supportive of hard work and determination to improve oneself. When you get your body in great shape, you will reap the rewards, but he will also be much happier and your relationship will blossom.

9. *All-Star Foods and Liquid Fuel*

We recommend the foods below for you to continue your daily strides at home and to improve your physical and mental wellness.

- **salads**-(w/ mushrooms, cucumbers, chick peas, peppers, olives, spinach w/ olive oil & balsamic vinegar), **rye bread**
- **couscous, barley**
- **citrus fruits (grapefruit, orange,)**-helps boost immune system
- **olive oil/flaxseed oil**-use these to cook the foods for your family; these healthy oils promote hormonal health
- **corn on the cob**-fuels body, helps prevent osteoporosis
- **steamed veggies**
- **berries (strawberries, blueberries, raspberries, cranberries, etc.)**-help prevent menstrual cramping & varicose/spider veins, balances hormones

High quality protein foods

- **egg whites** -easy, quick source of protein, they help slow the aging process
- **Luna bars, almonds, pumpkin seeds**
- **chicken breast**-supports hormonal health
- **fish, sushi**-helps the body's ability to withstand stress

Good sources of calcium

- low-fat yogurt
- cottage cheese
- veggie cheese
- low-fat milk
- soymilk

High fiber foods

- Oatmeal
- 5/5 cereals
- beans (kidney, soy, pinto, navy)
- broccoli
- yams
- pitas

Liquid Fuel

100-120 oz. WATER daily!

Savor in some delicious (hot or cold) GREEN TEA!

HOT TIP:

#1

*If breastfeeding, eat one extra meal a day high in calcium (low-fat milk, cottage cheese).

#2

*When hungry with cravings, carry sugar free breath mints or gum (only 5 calories per piece).

#3

*When eating out, broiled, baked, or grilled foods are desirable. Also, have clear soup and be selective in the salad bar (stay away from toppings, creamy dressings, mayonnaise, butter).

8. Foods to Avoid

Here are select popular foods that you and your child(ren) should avoid for most of the week. Going out once a week or twice a month for a treat is fine, but avoid the following foods listed below on a daily basis.

> ➢ Fast food—they typically contain lower nutritive calories, larger % saturated fat
> ➢ Local ice cream shoppe sweets
> ➢ Pizza, chips, cookies, soda, nachos, cheeseburgers
> ➢ Chocolate chip pancakes, high sugar cereals
> ➢ Chocolate, chocolate, chocolate! (avoid excessive amounts, moderation is the key)
> ➢ High G.I. carbs (ex. fruit juices, white bread, white pasta-contains refined flours)-consuming these often stimulate further hunger creating a vicious cycle of over-consumption
> ➢ Fried chicken, chicken paramigiana, meatball subs, bacon, sausage, pepperoni

HOT TIP:

#1

*Limit/avoid caffeinated beverages to prevent from unnecessary calcium losses.

7. Meals: How many & when?

It is important for you to heed this advice: EAT BREAKFAST! Do not skip this all-important meal to begin your day. Many of the clients in the past that we have dealt with had decided to skip breakfast figuring that this was reducing the total caloric intake for the day. What ends up happening, though, is a late night binge by the television. By eating breakfast, you stimulate your digestive system into action early on resulting in an increased metabolism throughout the duration of the entire day. Binging late at night causes the excess calories to be stored in your body as fat (your metabolism is slower at night). We can not stress enough the importance of eating breakfast daily.

TIPS TO REMEMBER:
-Eat every 3-4 hours after breakfast
-Limit what you eat late in the day
-Eat smallest meal late in the day (ex. salad with chicken breast and olive oil/vinegar)
-Let your husband indulge if he so chooses
-Eat a yogurt & fruit before working out on those early morning days

Here's the breakdown:

Workout days

6:30 A.M.	Fruit and yogurt
7:00 A.M.	Workout
8:30 A.M.	Fruit and yogurt
11:00 A.M.	moderate sized meal
2:00 P.M.	moderate sized meal
5:00 P.M.	small meal
7:30 P.M.	small meal

Non-workout days

7 A.M.	breakfast
10 A.M.	moderate sized meal
1 P.M.	moderate sized meal
4 P.M.	smaller sized meal
7 P.M.	smallest meal

6. *Supplementation & Sleep*

Depending on your child's sleeping patterns, your sleep may be fragmented throughout the nighttime. To help offset your lack of consistent sleep, try to take a nap while your child naps. Strive to obtain 7 hours of sleep a night.

What supplements are right for you?
    <u>A List</u>

    1. calcium (1500 mg)
    2. multivitamin (high in vitamin D, K & calcium)
    3. flaxseed oil (1000 mg capsules)

    <u>B List</u>

    1. ginkgo biloba
    2. melatonin

5. *Resistance Training* (◊ TOP TEN TOPICS, does lifting weights build muscle in women)
If you have no one to watch your child during your exercise session, bring your child to a health club/gym that has a well-supervised daycare center.

DURATION:
> 40 minute workout that will hit all of the key body parts
> 3 days a week: Monday, Wednesday, Friday

TEAMWORK:
> Workout w/ a friend that has a young child. You will have fun motivating each other during the workout, not to mention the daily gossip and what happened on Desperate Housewives.

A workout right for you!
- TOTAL BODY WORKOUT
- 3 sets of each exercise
- 15 repetitions (75% failure)
- 1 minute rest in between sets

1) Leg press
2) Machine chest press
3) Lying leg curl
4) Ball squats against the wall
5) Lying tricep dumbbell extensions
6) Dumbbell bicep curls
7) Lat rows
8) Crunches on stability ball

HOT BODY PARTS
$$$ *Triceps* $$$

A woman's body makeup stores fat here fairly easily. This is an important body part to keep toned for your body strength and the daily activities of picking up and moving things.
*An extra exercise that you can perform once a week:
-STANDING TRICEP EXTENSIONS

$$$ *Hamstrings & low back*$$$

Tight, weak hamstrings lead to a tight, weak low back. After carrying a child around in the womb for 9 months, your hamstrings and lower back have taken a toll. Let's counter this with some routines to regain your strength and flexibility in these areas.
-STRETCH AFTER EVERY WORKOUT (touch toes, slight bend in
knees, steady stretch without bouncing)
-SUPERMANS (15 times right before bed)
-YOGA & PILATES

$$$*Buttocks, hips, inner thighs*$$$

Unfortunately, the bad news is that you store fat here quite readily, too. The good news is that you are aware of it now and you can do something about it. Accompanying the leg press also try the following:
-3 SETS, 15 BALLET SQUATS-once a week in workout*
-3 SETS, WALKING LUNGES-try for 15 steps each leg*
*Alternate these two exercises each week

4. *Cardiovascular training* (⚡ TOP TEN TOPICS, is spot reducing possible)
After you have completed resistance training for the day (Mon/Wed/Fri), your body will dip into its fat storage more readily for fuel when doing a cardiovascular workout. Perform 20 minutes of moderately intense (65-75% max heart rate throughout) aerobic training to burn an optimal amount of fat calories. Our all-star choice for a supreme workout is the elliptical x-trainer. This machine does not put any stress on the joints. This truly is a great total body workout as it helps work your upper body along with your lower body.

During good weather days, you can take the pet and your child for a nice walk to get some fresh air. You will be benefiting you, your child and your pet. You can do some outdoor activities that will keep your body active while your child gets to release some energy and have a good time. It's a win-win situation!

3. *Sports*

This is a fun way to get out and socialize with some friends and burn some calories in the process. Try to engage in these activities a couple more times in addition to your aerobic training (20 min.) workouts during the week.

Enjoy some fun, yet intense whole body activities.
- Kick-boxing classes
- Spinning classes
- Yoga & Pilates (1 class an hour a week will do wonders for your SUPER HEALTH)
- Swimming/water aerobics

YOUR WEEKLY PLANNER:

3 DAYS: Mon/Wed/Fri = Resistance training + Cardio training

1 DAY: Tue or Thur = Yoga or Pilates

1 DAY: Any day = 1 hour enjoying your favorite class/sport

2. *How to Move More*   Activity level   5.5

"Moving back and forth around the house" tips

- Perform fun activities with your children that involve "movement" (playground, swimming, hiking, walking, yard work).
- Set an allotted time aside to watch a favorite TV show or play a favorite computer game vs. staying inside all day in front of the tube.
- Take the stairs whenever possible.
- Park as far away from stores when you go shopping.

1. *Obstacles and Ways To Conquer Them*

1. Staying disciplined working out	Three hours a week first thing in the morning should not be too difficult. If so, find a time where you can be consistent. Train with a partner to keep up motivation levels (for the both of you).
2. Monthly ups & downs	There may be some times (menstrual cycles) during the month when you are just not yourself & you crave goodies. We recom-

mend you feed those cravings. One or two bad days will not affect you if you get back on a consistent track for the rest of the month of eating and training right.

3. Proper food intake

Children, in general, love fast foods and foods high in sugar. Treat them once a week, but **you** don't need to eat those foods. Instead, choose salads & low-fat frozen yogurt. Remember, your children are always watching you. Lead by example and eat the all-star foods prescribed for you!

	Activity Level	Stress Level
	4.0	6.5

19. TRAVEL ✈

It's part of the job!

DRIVERS:

Driving for 12-16 hours a day can pose some different scenarios. It can be quite lonely at times with just you and the radio. Traffic issues can become stressful throughout your trip. Sitting for long periods can become boring and often times smoking & consuming various stimulants to stay awake are sometimes the unfortunate answers to these long, tedious trips. Concentration on the road is always a must, especially operating such a large vehicle. Going long distances requires taking breaks to eat & those truck stop buffets can be an unhealthy resort for food.

FLYERS:

You are dealing with a different cast of people each day, but with the same intent: to serve their needs. Whether it is to stay focused for the responsibility of many people's lives (piloting the plane), or to assist in other duties to help passengers (stewards/stewardesses, etc.), your job is important and requires being on planes for long extended periods. Airplane food, jet lag, and dehydration are some terms that go along with your profession. Air travel can also present some unique challenges.

10. *Lifestyle Tips*

DRIVERS:

Staying alert at all times while driving is a huge responsibility on top of getting to your destination on time. By eating soundly on a daily basis, this will help you stay alert and is much healthier as compared to relying on stimulants (such as caffeine) to keep you awake.

Carry a set of dumbbells and a jump rope in your truck. So when you feel sluggish throughout your trip, pull over and exercise for 5 minutes to stimulate your body in a healthy, beneficial manner to get the blood flowing. You don't even have to wait until you feel tired. If you have the time, pull over every 2-3 hours. It's amazing what you can do for your body WHILE WORKING!

Sit up tall while driving. Having good posture is crucial, especially if you consistently take long trips. Listen to motivational tapes and quality music. Do not eat at truck stop buffets. Instead, stop at supermarkets that are right off the highway and pick up some all-star foods there (enough to keep you going for your time spent on the road).

FLYERS:

From time to time, take note of how most Europeans and Asians appear physically. Their lifestyles and activity levels certainly contrast the "American lifestyle". Sit up tall with good posture while flying. When not flying, move around. Work out before your flights (domestic-home gyms; international-hotel gyms). Eat frequently and bring your food with you at all times.

Drink plenty of water. The cabin increases fluid losses due to the high- pressure environment so water consumption is of the utmost importance. Dehydration is often a byproduct of flying. If you aren't a member of the airplane staff or part of the piloting team, then take advantage of the flight and get some work done.

9. *All-Star Foods and Liquid Fuel*

FOODS AT WORK

➤ Grilled chicken breast on rye bread, apple, water (16 oz.)
➤ All-star snacks: carrot sticks, pears, dried prunes, raisins, sunflower seeds, Brazil nuts, Clif bars, Pure Protein bars, water
➤ Low-fat cheese products, low-fat yogurt, cottage cheese, soymilk, low-fat milk, water
➤ Meal replacements & shakers

NOTE: It is very important to have these foods with you when flying because you can not stop to pick up something half way into a trip (like truck drivers can). Also, airport foods can be expensive and there are very few healthy choices. Lastly, don't go anywhere without that 24 oz. water bottle.

FOODS AT HOME/HOTEL

➤ Egg whites, multi-grain toast, orange juice, grapefruit, green tea
➤ Oatmeal, whole grain cereals (following 5/5 rule), water
➤ Gardenburgers, soyburgers, mushroom kabobs, chicken soup, corn on the cob, beans (baked, kidney, lima, soy)
➤ ean ground beef, top round sirloin (delivers oxygen to muscles & energizes), sweet potato, mixed veggies
➤ Low glycemic carbs, monounsaturated fats, quality lean proteins
  • Roasted turkey breast on pumpernickel bread, peanuts
  • Salads w/ shrimp, chickpeas, leafy veggies, broccoli, olive oil & vinegar
  • Grilled fish (salmon, swordfish) w/ ½ tbsp. flaxseed oil cooked on it, brown rice, asparagus
  • Chicken breast w/ ½ tbsp. olive oil, whole wheat pasta, mushrooms
  • Try to drink 1 gallon of water daily

HOT TIP:
#1 (for drivers)

*You have a great amount of control over the actions during your day: when you eat, drink, and sleep. When you stop to eat something, choose **healthy** choices. It may be easy to stop at a truck stop, fuel up and grab a quick snack there. Your choices here are crucial to your SUPER HEALTH and how well the remainder of your trip will go (energy-wise).

#2 (for flyers)

*Airlines do not always provide low-fat meals. However, low-fat or vegetarian meals are sometimes available if requested. You do not want to take this chance. Play it smart and bring your all-star food selections!

8. Foods to Avoid
   DRIVERS:
   ➤ **Truck stop buffets**
      - You can consume heavy portions all at once. On top of that, these foods are high in fats & preservatives.
   ➤ **Fast food, convenience store foods**
   ➤ **High glycemic quick hits:** soda, graham crackers, candy, chips, granola bars, fruit juice

   FLYERS:
   ➤ **Caffeine:** coffee, café mochas. café lattes, soda, etc.
      - Caffeine will dehydrate you (a diuretic). In order to remain hydrated while drinking caffeinated beverages, you would have to drink 16 oz. of water for every 8 oz. of coffee consumed.

   OTHER FOODS TO AVOID:
   ➤ Muffins, donuts, light & sweet flavored coffee, cookies, bagels
   ➤ Chinese food, deli meats, bread
   ➤ Pasta, white rice, white flour products (1st ingredient is enriched flour-do not buy)
   ➤ Avoid alcoholic beverages (increase risk of dehydration, loss of alertness)
   ➤ "Fatty" dinners: pork, macaroni & cheese, eggplant parmigiana, penne ala vodka, pizza w/ the works

7. Meals: How many & when?
   Consume small meals frequently throughout the day (every 3 hours). Make breakfast your biggest meal of the day. Eating every 3 hours will also help relieve boredom. It will give you something (healthy) to do.

It is the healthiest and longest lasting way to keep your energy levels high (unlike a pot of coffee/popping pills daily).

Portion your meals so you don't over-consume all at once. This feeling of being extremely full will deprive a good amount of oxygen supply to your brain, resulting in a feeling of lethargy. Remember, this will exacerbate the sluggish feeling for individuals in your profession due to the extensive period of sitting/inactivity while driving or flying.

6. *Supplementation & Sleep*

Sleep may be either interrupted, in varying time zones, or you simply may not be able to sleep from traveling so much. Try to average 7 hours a night of sleep on the plane for passengers. If you work on the plane and cannot sleep while flying, you must average 7 hrs a sleep a night, especially because you may be traveling through different time zones and neglecting sleep will definitely catch up to you when you least expect it. Drivers, take powernaps of 10-15 minutes during the day on your road trips (when not driving-of course!). These naps will recharge your batteries. Whatever you do, do NOT neglect sleep trying to get to your destination quicker. This will just wear you out even more. You control how far you go and when ever possible, rest to get those indispensable z's in!

What supplements are right for you?
   <u>A List</u>

   1. multivitamin
   2. antioxidant
   3. melatonin
   4. ZMA
   5. tyrosine
   6. vitamin B (100-200 mg)

   <u>**B** List</u>

   1. ginkgo
   2. ginseng
   3. caffeine

NOTE: Avoid ephedra, or any other powerful stimulant. It's not healthy & potentially very dangerous. Xenadrine EFX & other ephedra-free products are better choices, but still have potential health risks. Consult your physician first.

5. *Resistance Training* (✈ TOP TEN TOPICS, proper form)

Focus on the weekly goals. Because of your intense traveling schedule, getting three days a week of quality workouts will be fine rather than worrying about daily workouts. Your workouts will occupy 3 hours out of the week.

When you are on the road, find gyms nearby or workout at your hotel gym. The fees are relatively inexpensive for working out for the day ($5-$10 range) as compared to purchasing a six-pack of beer, 2 packs of cigarettes and a box of donuts.

TRUCK DRIVERS:

- Heavy, compound movements
- Total body workouts
- 3 days a week
- For each exercise, perform 1 warm up set (12-15 repetitions) followed by 2 working sets (6-8 repetitions)

A workout right for you!

- **Do this workout 3 days a week and see the results!**

  1) Bench press
  2) Squats
  3) Seated lat rows
  4) Seated military press (dumbbells or barbells)
  5) Stiff-leg deadlifts
  6) Barbell curls
  7) 50 crunches

FLYERS:

Due to prolonged periods of inactivity, we need to get your body moving. Find a gym on the road in between flights to workout.

- Circuit training workouts
- 3 days a week
- 3 total circuits
- 15 second rest between exercises
- 2 minute rest between circuits

A workout right for you!

- FEMALES: 12-15 reps; 75-85% failure on last 2 reps
- MALES: 8-12 reps; 80-90% failure on last 2 reps

CIRCUIT #1

1) 25 bodyweight squats
2) machine chest press
3) seated leg press
4) machine shoulder press
5) lying leg curl
6) preacher curl
7) seated lat row
8) hanging leg raises
9) standing tricep extensions (2 ropes)

CIRCUIT #2

REPEAT CIRCUIT #1

CIRCUIT #3

REPEAT CIRCUIT #1

HOT TIP: (truckers)
#1

*Carry a pair of 25 lb. dumbbells with you in your truck. You can perform the workout below anytime & anywhere (in the case that you can't get to a gym). If you feel ambitious, you can get in a couple of extra workouts. Just pull out those weights at a rest area and get going. Perform 2 to 3 sets of each exercise below of 10 repetitions.

1) shrugs
2) squat thrusts
3) stationary lunges
4) shoulder presses
5) 1-arm rows

6) lying chest press
7) bicep curls
8) 2-minute jumping jacks

HOT TIP: (flyers)
#1

*In case you can't find a gym to workout at (ex. if the hotel you are staying at doesn't have one), hit the local park and perform an exercise that is a total body workout, WEIGHT-FREE!

1) 2 minutes-jumping jacks
2) 1 minute-shadow boxing
3) 40-50 pushups
4) 25 squats
5) 30 crunches
6) 25 supermans
7) repeat #1-6 twice for a great, outdoor workout

4. *Cardiovascular training*
   ❑ **3 days a week, 15 minutes after weight training**
   ❑ **HR steady 75-80% for 15 minutes**
   ❑ **Different modes:**
      • Day 1: precor elliptical
      • Day 2: treadmill
      • Day 3: stairmaster

No gym available?

Day 1: 15 minute jog (try to do 2 miles in this timeframe)

Day 2: 10 wind sprints for 50 yards on a track or at a park for 50 yards

Day 3: Shadow box (2 minutes)
Jumping jacks (2 minutes)
Shadow box (2 minutes)
Jumping jacks (2 minutes)
Jog for 1 mile

3. *Sports*
Active, whole-body activities are encouraged when home.

- Tennis
- Pilates
- Golf
- Racquetball
- Cross-country skiing
- Hiking

HOT TIP (while traveling):
#1

*Drivers, carry a basketball somewhere in your cab. When you are on the road, you can go to a local park & shoot some hoops. If you enjoy mountain biking or rollerblading instead, bring those along for your pleasures.

#2

*Flyers, take aerobic classes at a gym near your hotel. Take a comforting swim at the pool in the hotel.

2. *How to Move More*   <u>Activity level</u>   <u>4.0</u> (✈ TOP TEN TOOLS, especially #9, move more)

DRIVERS:

When driving for long periods of time, find a rest stop (every 1-2 hours) and instead of purchasing a pick-me-up cup of coffee, keep your money in your wallet and perform 50 jumping jacks. Then, finish with a nice stretch of touching your toes and holding for 10 seconds, then reaching for the sky for 10 seconds alternating this great stretch back and forth a few times. This will do absolute wonders for your mood & alertness on the road. Keep a pair of handgrips in the car and squeeze them intermittently during your trip (especially when you are stuck in a traffic jam). This helps as a stress-buster relieving tension in negative situations.

FLYERS:

For long, intensified sitting periods, you are recommended to get up every hour (if possible) and take a walk to the back of the cabin, stretch, touch your toes and then touch the skies, then perform 10 squats.

Perform these on the hour (ex. 3-hour flight- 3 times, 9-hour flight-9 times). Monitor your posture each hour, too.

If you are working overseas or across the nation, walking from airport to taxi, transporting your luggage will keep you moving. Take the stairs in the hotel. Enjoy your new surroundings and take in the fresh air & new daily adventures.

1. *Obstacles and Ways To Conquer Them*

DRIVERS

1. Driving & sitting alone	Stay motivated by listening to motivational tapes to keep your spirits high. Spend this time to learn another language. You never know when you'll need it in your daily travels. Stop every 1-2 hours for a break. You are the boss. Many times you may feel that you are behind the 8-ball and you need to keep going and going. Five minutes will not kill you, but actually benefit you greatly. Stay motivated and train 3 times a week. Know your routes and where to stop to pick up your all-star foods and toworkout.
2. Eating soundly and staying alert	Anticipate your needs on the road. Plan ahead on when you are going to pick up your all-star foods for the day. This will save you time and money in the long run. For you, time is money. You may be driving for 16 hours a day (some may go for greater time intervals) to get the shipments delivered in a timely manner. You are very important and appreciated in what you do. If it weren't for you, other businesses would not receive their desired goods, which ultimately would not come to its purchasers (us)!
3. When & where to workout	The importance of having a plan can not be over-stressed here. For instance, if you are going on an 8-day delivery trip, you want to plan your workouts, rest area breaks, sleep schedule, where to get your all-star foods, while still getting your deliveries done on time. Set yourself up for success professionally and physically through preparation! Carry plenty of water with you at all times.

FLYERS

1. Sitting on airplanes

You want to avoid dehydration when flying, which increases the effects of jetlag. Have a 24 oz. container of water by your side at all times and drink up. Get out of your seat on the hour. Refer to our "moving more" tips to keep everything working properly.

2. Staying alert and focused (pilots)

Being responsible for so many lives on a daily basis is quite a stressful undertaking. The program that we have designed for you will further enhance your mentality & physicality. Eat and bring the recommended all-star foods with you. Find those workout facilities at your destinations and your body will respond with great passion!

3. Where & when to workout

Again, set your priorities straight. Sit down at the beginning of your week and plan your 3 weekly workouts. Don't let yourself down! Obtain your 3-workouts a week goal for 2 months and in no time, it will become a lifestyle habit!

	Activity Level	Stress Level
	2.0	6.5

20. WHITE-COLLAR EMPLOYEES (males) 🍵

It's part of the job!

It's a fact that you may not be getting as much physical activity throughout the workweek as you would like. On top of that, your stress level can be peaked at times. You may find yourself, in large part, sitting throughout the day.

Your profession requires a great deal of mental exercise. You are indeed getting a strenuous mental work-out during the week. This mental fatigue can take a toll on your physical wellness. Many times you are trapped in a room where fresh air may be lacking and your body's fuel tank is running low. These long hours at the office can lead to mental burnout if there isn't some form of a healthy outlet.

10. *Lifestyle Tips* (🍵 TOP TEN TOOLS, especially #9, move more)

Eating properly and frequently are two fundamental tips vital to your success. Try and prepare most of your foods at home. Ask your wife (if possible) to help. I'm sure with all of the efforts that you put in throughout a day's work that she would be glad to help you. Then, bring these foods to work.

Exercise in the morning throughout the workweek. This will give you sustained energy throughout the day and prevent from over-exhausting the brain. You will even accomplish more during the day due to your increased mental and physical strength. In addition, your metabolism will be elevated and your body will be functioning at an optimal speed. Many of you young bucks may enjoy engaging in weekend sports. With proper exercise throughout the week, you will be enjoying the weekends and feel adequately prepared for the following workweek.

Use your multi-tasking ability to develop a strong work ethic and self-discipline for your own SUPER HEALTH. At work, stay active on the hour, even if you get up and take a walk to get some water to drink or get up to go to use the restroom. The key factor here is that you are moving!

9. *All-Star Foods and Liquid Fuel*

FOODS AT WORK

Low G.I. carbohydrates

apples	all-bran cereal
pears	low-fat yogurt
wheat pitas	old-fashioned oatmeal

<u>Low G.I. meat alternatives</u>

gardenburger
soyburger
low-fat beef patties (90% fat-free)

If you didn't bring your lunch, pick up one of these healthy choices:

1) Grilled chicken breast salad w/ olive oil, balsamic vinegar, broccoli, cucumbers, celery, spinach, olives, tomatoes, & a whole egg cut up
                    OR
2) Tuna sushi & california rolls

<u>High quality all star snacks</u>

Clif bars   Luna bars
Kashi Go-Lean bars   Pure Protein bars
chicken soup

Liquid Fuel

Always have water by your desk!! Get a 20 oz. bottle and fill it up 6 times a day (=120 oz)

Additional goodie: GREEN TEA (hot or cold)

FOODS AT HOME

whole-grain cereals (low-GI quality carbs to fuel the muscles)
w/ soymilk/low-fat milk
NOTE: Use the 5/5 rule (fiber content in cereal should equal at least 5
grams or more and sugar content should be less than 5 grams)
grilled top round sirloin steak, asparagus, couscous
grilled chicken breast, brown rice, zucchini, mushroom kabobs
grilled salmon w/ lemon, sweet potato, split pea soup
egg white omelette w/ kidney beans, veggie cheese/low-fat
cheese, broccoli, spinach

HOT TIP:
#1

*A healthy choice to use when cooking would be olive oil and flaxseed oil. Add some hot sauce (speeds up the metabolism) on some of the all-star food choices. Montreal chicken seasoning and steak seasoning will add a great amount of flavor to your foods.

#2

*Drink decaffeinated beverages 95% of the time.

8. Foods to Avoid

A) <u>Vending machine foods</u>

soda, chips, cookies, candy

B) <u>Foods cooked in heavy oil, fried foods</u>

macaroni & cheese	**pizza**
meatball grinders	**nachos**

NOTE: Excessive quantities of olive oil is not healthy.

C) <u>Frozen food entrees</u>

high in sodium, fat, & preservatives

D) <u>Caffeine</u>

Best in moderation, best if consumed before training (200 mg/med./black) Use honey & soymilk as opposed to cream & sugar

E) <u>All refined carbs</u>

white rice   crackers   chips   rice cakes

F) Other temptations

pasta (esp. after 8 P.M.)
sausage/bacon & homefries for breakfast
double bacon cheeseburger, French fries, milkshake
dark turkey meat, stuffing, pumpkin pie, cranberry sauce, biscuits
New England clam chowder, fried shrimp, clams w/ melted butter

HOT TIP:
#1

* Refrain from consuming those late night drinks to take the edge off. If you are working out consistently and eating right throughout the day, then your body and mind will already be in the right place.

7. Meals: How many & when? (TOP TEN TOPICS-glycemic index)
*Training days
Upon waking up in the morning, prepare a meal replacement shake with bananas & strawberries. Before you go to workout, drink half of the shake. Upon completing your workout, consume the remaining half.

Eat smaller meals from the all-star food choices making certain that you include a mix of quality protein and quality carbohydrates (low G.I.) with each meal. Eat every 3 hours or so throughout the day up until around 8 P.M.

Here's the breakdown:

7 A.M.	½ meal replacement
9 A.M.	½ meal replacement
11 A.M.	meal
2 P.M.	meal/snack
5 P.M.	meal
7:30 P.M.	smallest meal/snack

*Non-training days

7 A.M.	meal
10 A.M.	meal/snack
1 P.M.	meal
4 P.M.	meal
7 P.M.	smallest meal/snack

* Schedule may be different for each profession, but sequence and intervals are the same.

HOT TIP:
#1

*Decrease your carbohydrate intake as the day progresses. Consume the most in the morning and the least at night.

#2

*Eating 4-6 small meals throughout the day will crank up your metabolism.

6. Supplementation & Sleep

The recommended 8 hours a day holds true for you guys! Your schedule in the gym and at work will demand optimum energy. The daily stresses take a toll physically and mentally. Do not sacrifice sleep during the week and figure that you will redeem your losses on the weekend. You will bottom out at 70% of your peak potential most of the time. This is not conducive for maintaining or developing muscle tone.

What supplements are right for you?
A List

1. meal replacement
2. multivitamin/multimineral
3. antioxidants- help fight free radicals, which are a byproduct of intense exercise and an intense, stressful profession (high in vitamin C & E)
4. vitamin B (100 mg)

B List

1. ZMA
2. melatonin
3. ginseng, tyrosine, ginkgo stack
4. caffeine (pre-training-200 mg)
5. creatine/glutamine

5. Resistance Training
Two words: SHORT, INTENSE
Three days: Monday, Wednesday, Friday (mornings)
Duration: 40-45 minutes
Type of training: CIRCUIT (total-3 circuits including your whole body)

> ➤ 40-45 minutes of circuit training will burn approximately 600 calories
> ➤ includes a series of exercises in sequence without rest in between sets
> ➤ the goal is to keep your heart rate at 55%-60% during each circuit
>
> NOTE: You can buy a polar h.r. monitor to wear around your chest.
>
> ➤ good way to overload metabolic system
> ➤ great way to reach higher levels of fitness

A workout right for you!
- Perform a full circuit 3 times with 2 minutes rest in between each circuit
- Do not rest between the exercises within the circuit
- GENTLEMEN: 8-12 repetitions; 90% failure on last 2-3 reps

HOT TIP:
#1

*This workout will be beneficial for both burning fat calories at an elevated rate and stimulating your muscle tone while you are sitting at your desk.

Circuit #1
1) 50-100 jumping jacks
2) machine chest press
3) lat pulldowns
4) dumbbell bicep curls
5) standing tricep pulldowns
6) leg press
7) lying leg curls
8) stationary lunges
9) hanging leg raises

REST FOR TWO MINUTES

Circuit #2
Repeat circuit #1 and rest for two minutes.

Circuit #3
Repeat circuit #1.

HOT BODY PARTS
$$$ Hamstrings & lower back $$$

Your job requires a great deal of sitting, talking on the telephone, and working on the computer throughout the day. Stretch your hamstrings after working out and during the day. Before you go to bed, perform 20 supermans by raising your legs and arms up at the same time while lying face down on the ground, holding that position for 3 seconds.

4. Cardiovascular training

After you have completed resistance training for the day (Mon/Wed/Fri), perform 15 minutes of fairly intense aerobic training. Keep your heartrate between 70-75% of your max heart rate throughout the cardio session. Choose between the elliptical x-trainer, stepmill, or the treadmill. The key here is to use a mode that gets you up off your gluteus and will incorporate your whole body.

On one of your days off from training (Tue or Thur), take your lunch break and get out of the office to walk for 45 minutes to an hour. Focus on walking with your shoulders back and keeping your chest high. Use your ipod and enjoy some tunes while you take in some fresh air.

The weekend is here! Here is a great, challenging workout that you can do on the weekend and if you enjoy playing sports competitively, this workout will help you at any sport you enjoy competing in!

Here is a 15 minute plyometric power/interval training session sure to keep you moving!
- 1 minute-jump rope
- 2 sets-25 jump squats
- 2 minutes-step ups on an 18-inch step (holding hands overhead, alternating legs)
- 1 minute-jump rope
- 2 sets-25 jump squats
- 2 minutes-treadmill (6.5 speed, 6.0 incline)
- 1 minute-jump rope
- 2 minutes-treadmill (6.5 speed, 6.5 incline)
- 3 minutes-treadmill cool down (3.6 speed)

HOT TIP:
#1

*Try to incorporate this workout into your schedule twice a month on the weekends.
You will notice immense gains in speed, explosiveness & power!

3. *Sports*

This is a fun way to compete and burn calories. Sports that you would benefit from would be whole body athletic activities.

Enjoy some great whole body activities (especially on the weekends)
- Basketball (leagues, YMCA, open gyms)
- Flag football leagues
- Softball
- Volleyball
- Road races
- Bodybuilding
- Yoga & Pilates-gets the body in proper alignment and keeps muscles long and supple (after hours in a stagnant position)
- Golf-walk rather than ride and take in nature's finest qualities

2. *How to Move More*   <u>Activity level</u>   <u>2.0</u>

It is all about getting your body moving throughout the day. Your profession requires less movement during the day than many other professions (ex. builders, electricians, mailmen, policemen, wait staff, etc.). These tips of how to move more will greatly complement the other tips that you have implemented into your daily/weekly schedule.

"The movers and the shakers" tips

- Set a timer of some sort (ex. watch, beeper, computer) to remind you on the hour that it is time to get up and move around.
- Go outside and get some fresh air 1 hour.
- Perform 10 bodyweight squats the next hour.
- Stretch arms overhead and then to the floor the next hour.
- Take the stairs everywhere you go. Skip steps if you are really ambitious.
- Be daring! Buy a stability ball and bring it into work (yes in front of all of your co-workers) and use it as a chair! This act of bravery will pay off with improved posture and an additional burning of approx. 200 calories a day. You will be recruiting many different muscle groups to help you keep balanced and stay upright.

1. *Obstacles and Ways To Conquer Them*

1.Skipping meals at work   With your profession, you may become tied down for hours on end without realizing that you haven't eaten. Bring and keep your all-star food selections by you at all times. Have the alarm go off every 3 hours to notify you that it's time to fuel up.

2. High stress level at times

Take it outside guys! Get some fresh air for a while. Stay consistent w/ proper training and eating. At home, try to focus on anything other than work.

3. Finding time to workout

Workout first thing in the morning. This will get you in a good routine and develop good habits. Being that early bird is the spark that will light your fire throughout the day setting you up for success. Energy levels will be sustained for longer durations and will be higher throughout the day. In turn, this will benefit your.resistance training sessions and .you will see amazing results.

4. Sitting down all day

Find a reason (any reason) to get up. Get something to drink. Go to the restroom. Just keep on moving! Use our tips mentioned and keep moving!

CHAPTER 7

TOP TEN FIT FAST FOODS

We realize how it is for you during your busy workweek. You may not have time each day to prepare an ideal "all-star" meal. We provide some alternatives that will please the palette with a deliciously healthy meal. Here are some recommended fast foods that you can choose from that pack a healthy punch!

BOSTON MARKET

	CALORIES	CARBS	PROTEIN	FAT
1.1/4 WHITE CHICKEN (no skin and wing)	170	2	33	4
RICE PILAF	140	24	2	4
STEAMED VEGGIES	30	6	2	0
1 HONEY WHEAT ROLL	130	19	2	2
TOTAL	470	51	39	10
2. SKINLESS TURKEY BREAST	170	1	36	1
BUTTERNUT SQUASH	150	25	2	6
GREEN BEANS	70	6	1	4
1 HONEY WHEAT ROLL	130	19	2	2
TOTAL	520	51	41	13
3. HONEY-GLAZED HAM	210	10	24	8

DILL NEW POTATO	130	25	3	2
FRESH FRUIT	70	16	1	0
1 HONEY WHEAT ROLL	130	19	2	2
TOTAL	540	70	30	12

MCDONALDS

4. EGG MCMUFFIN	300	29	18	12
12 OZ. ORANGE JUICE	120	28	0	0
TOTAL	420	57	18	12
5. GRILLED CHIX/COBB SALAD	270	9	33	11
NEWMAN'S COBB DRESSING	120	9	1	9
TOTAL	390	18	34	20

WENDY'S

6. GRILLED CHIX SANDWICH (W/REDUCED CAL. HONEY MUSTARD, TOMATO, LETTUCE, SAND WICH BUN)	300	36	24	6
TOTAL	300	36	24	6
7. PLAIN BAKED POTATO	300	70	7	0
SMALL CHILI	200	21	17	6
SIDE SALAD (OIL+VINEGAR)	105	7	2	5
TOTAL	505	98	31	11

SUBWAY

8. 6" TURKEY BREAST (STANDARD VEGGIES, WHEAT ROLL)	280	46	18	5
TOTAL	280	46	18	5
9. 6" DOUBLE MEAT CHIX (STANDARD VEGGIES, WHEAT ROLL)	430	50	38	8
TOTAL	430	50	38	8

DUNKIN DONUTS

10. 1 PLAIN WHEAT BAGEL	280	48	8	2
16 OZ. LOWFAT MILK	220	52	16	2
1 MED. COFFEE (w/ Splenda)	0	0	0	0
TOTAL	500	100	24	4

THESE ARE FIT FAST FOODS THAT YOU CAN GET ON THE GO FOR BREAKFAST, LUNCH OR DINNER.

CHAPTER 8

TOP TEN TOPICS

1. Calories A Person Burns Daily

Our society today is plagued by the increasing "need for speed". We are living on the information super-highway with fashions and trends being set and returning from years past. Following the fitness and exercise path, many "revolutionary" diets have come to the rescue including "The Atkins Diet", "The South Beach Diet", "The Mediterranean Diet", "The Makers Diet" and also "Dr. Phil's Plan". These diets have noble intentions to help people achieve a more sleek physique. Why people diet and what method they use is heavily determined by cultural trends. We are living in a fast paced society often times a click away from our wants and needs being instantly satisfied.

An unwanted trend in our society

One very disappointing trend in our country that is rapidly becoming what many consider an epidemic is obesity. Two-thirds of Americans are overweight (body wt. heavier than normal for age/height). Half of these individuals are considered obese, which includes over 60 million people nationwide. If society is trending in this direction, what can we do to help ourselves? We need a viable solution, right? An answer to fix it all is what we are in search of. More appropriately, we need the FACTS. The reality behind much of this weight increase is *we eat more and move less.*

Many U.S. citizens have a sedentary lifestyle and burn an average of 14 calories/lb. a day without induced activity. The fact is that eating more than this level will create a positive caloric intake where energy intake is greater than energy expenditure resulting in a weight gain over time. The opposite is true for negative caloric balance where energy expenditure is greater than energy intake.

The bottom line fact to underscore here is that if you like to eat, then you need to MOVE MORE. From the following chart, locate where you fit in. Which activities interest you and determine the number of calories that you would like to burn. You can set up a daily/weekly schedule following the tips mentioned to track your success. Move more than you eat and you will accomplish the feat!

Activity	Calories burned/hour
Bicycling (8 mph)	330
Bicycling (15 mph)	612
Walking (3 mph)	270
Walking briskly (5 mph)	440
Jogging (6 mph)	655
Golf (w/ a cart)	200
Golf (w/out a cart)	320
Gardening	220
Tennis	450
Hiking	490
Bowling	270
Swimming	310
Circuit Training	750
Basketball	780

2. Glycemic Index

Searching in the Sunday newspaper for that "low carb diet" of the week seems to be a popular trend nowadays. Knowing the facts about carbohydrates and how to moderate your diet will lead you on the road to SUPER HEALTH.

How does the G.I. rating system work?

The glycemic index (G.I.) rating system ranks foods accordingly. It is your best guide to choosing smart carbohydrates. The G.I. is a 20-year old carbohydrate rating system that was developed in the early 1980s by University of Toronto researchers to help control diabetes. The G.I. ranks carbs by their effect on the blood sugar levels in the body. The G.I. assigns carb-containing foods a number that is based on how they affect one's blood sugar levels after the food is eaten.

For instance, foods with a G.I. rating below 60 cause a low rise in blood sugar levels. Foods between 60-75 raise levels a bit higher, while foods above 75 spike blood sugar levels rather quickly. This ranking system focuses largely on these carb-containing foods and their effects on our blood-sugar levels.

Low G.I. foods (under 55)-carbs broken down slowly & release glucose slow & steady into the bloodstream
Intermediate G.I. foods (55-75)-carbs broken down moderately releasing glucose a bit faster into the bloodstream
High G.I. foods (over 75)-carbs broken down quickly during digestion, glucose release is quickest and high

YOUR GOAL: 99% carbs eaten on a daily basis should be less than 75 G.I.

Under 55

Low-fat yogurt	15	Orange	44
Peanuts	16	Grapes	45
Soybeans	20	Bulgur	48
Green leafy veggies	20	Old-fashioned oatmeal	49
Grapefruit	25	(non-instant)	
Pearl barley	25	Canned baked beans	49
Kidney beans	27	Pumpernickel bread	51
Skim milk	30	Brown Rice	54
Soy milk	31		
Cherries	32		
Apple	38		
Whole wheat spaghetti	39		
Pear	39		
All-bran cereal	41		

Intermediate 55-75

Sweet potato	56	Grapenuts	65
Special K cereal	59	Banana 67	
Yam	60	Cheese pizza	68
White rice	61	Whole-wheat bread	70
Blueberry muffin	62	Carrots	71
Rye bread	63	White bread	72
Ice cream	64	Watermelon	73
Granola bar	65		

High 75+

Bagels	78	Jelly beans	89
Mashed potatoes	81	Pretzels	89
Bread-stuffing mix	82	French bread	91
Doughnuts	83	Rice cakes	93
French fries	84	Frozen yogurt	94
Baked potato	86	Cookies	101
Instant oatmeal	88		

What is the significance of the G.I.?

Carbohydrates are a major source of energy for the body providing four calories for each gram. Understand that carbohydrates in the form of glycogen (stored blood sugar (glucose) in the liver and muscle cells) form about 1% of all energy reserves. However, this small percentage is essential for support of central nervous system metabolism and for your fitness and wellness goals. They fuel our bodies for daily functions, sports & exercise, building and repairing muscle, and boosting energy levels. Now, you may say, what's the difference: a donut vs. a bagel. A carb is a carb, right? It is the "kind of carbs" that we eat to which we need to pay careful mind.

Just remember one word: LOW. If your goal is for SUPER HEALTH, wellness, or that peak physique, then you want to consume low-moderate GI carbs. One of the only times that your body should experience high-end GI carbs is directly after a workout session. It is at this specific instance that your muscles are depleted of glycogen and in need of this quick fix of sugar.

What are the results of eating high G.I. carbs all of the time?

One negative of high glycemic foods such as candy, cookies, and certain bread types is that they contain processed sugars. They lack the necessary nutrients that natural sugars such as fruits and vegetables contain.

Here is a second problem with eating high G.I. carbs. When you eat high G.I. carbs, your blood sugar soars and in response to that, the hormone insulin is secreted for duty. Insulin's job is to control this "sugar rush" by scooping up the excess glucose (sugar) and storing it in muscle tissue. However, if the muscle tissue is filled up with glycogen, then the insulin will have no choice but to deposit it into the dreaded adipose tissue (a.k.a. fat cells). We certainly want to stay clear of these high G.I. carbs unless they are directly consumed post-workout when the sugar has somewhere to go (to the muscle) other than to fat cells. Keep it LOW!

TOP 10 BENEFITS OF EATING LOW G.I. CARBS

10. *Contain a high-fiber content*

Carbohydrates supply many essential vitamins and minerals to our body, but also supply an important non-nutrient for a healthful diet: FIBER. Researchers have indicated the value of fiber and the role it contributes to a reduction in heart disease, cancer and diabetes. Fiber also contributes to an increase in one's metabolism throughout the day.

A person should try to consume about 30-40 grams of fiber daily, as it is essential to health and helps decrease body fat. Foods below a level of 75 contain a greater amount of fiber than higher G.I. foods. Fiber lowers insulin levels and absorbs water. Hence, the water will occupy more space in the body keeping you satiated for longer and promoting a more efficient running gastrointestinal tract.

9. *Helps in preventing/eliminating digestive complications*

Many digestive complications can be prevented through intake of these foods.

8. *Helps prevent cancer*

Low G.I. foods higher in fiber help to prevent many types of cancer such as colon, rectum and prostate cancer to name a few.

7. *Keeps a healthy heart*

Heart disease is the leading killer in America. This is due in large part to an over-consumption of many high G.I. carbs. The resulting insulin spikes delivered from your pancreas can take a toll. The heart is a muscle that works all the time at varying intensities. This muscle requires help from glycogen stores for short bursts in high intense activities. Your blood gets disturbed when sugar levels are frequently altered. In consuming these high G.I. carbs, the sugar rush can result in long-term damage to your heart.

6. *Helps prevent type II diabetes*

Diabetes is an autoimmune disease resulting in an unstable, higher than normal blood sugar level. This condition has reached epidemic levels in the U.S. More than 90% of all diabetics are non-insulin dependent/adult-onset (type II), which is prompted in large part by the sedentary American lifestyle. Type II can be and should be prevented through exercise and dietary control. If a person consumes low glycemic carbs, this will help for a slow and steady release of sugar throughout the bloodstream. Hence, the blood sugar level will remain more "homeostatic" (constant) preventing sharp spikes and declines in insulin levels. The low G.I. carbs are widely accepted as a strategy/solution for fighting diabetes in Canada and England.

5. *Kickstarts your metabolism*

Fiber is an animal in your body! As your body uses a tremendous amount of energy to break down and digest foods high in fiber, eating small, frequent meals containing fiber will help your metabolism to fire on all cylinders. The tamed beast inside will operate like a furnace devouring calories consistently throughout the day turning you into a lean machine.

4. *Helps you stay alert and fuels the brain*

Good morning sunshine! It's time for your daily dose of "low G.I. beauties". Why you ask? Low G.I. foods, especially when eaten at breakfast time, will increase alertness by fueling your brain with a steady supply of a needed sugar throughout the day. These low G.I. carbs will give you that mental edge throughout the day.

3. *Suppresses your appetite*

Stable blood sugar levels, which low G.I. foods promote, will keep you going strong for longer periods. These foods are more slowly absorbed, thus suppressing the appetite. You will not feel as tempted to open up the cabinet for that late night snack while you watch SportsCenter.

2. *Energizes you for longer*

Studies have shown that you will exercise longer and stronger after eating a low-G.I. meal compared to a high G.I. meal.

1. *Helps shed the unwanted pounds*

This ladies and gentlemen is the BOTTOM LINE! High levels of insulin are necessary for the body when we eat foods of a high G.I. rating (this should ideally be after a workout). Ninety percent of the day should be low G.I. carbs. Again, constant blood glucose levels keep you going for longer durations, which in turn suppress the appetite helping you to lose weight in a healthy, non-starving manner.

THE TRUTH ABOUT CARBS

Let the truth be told that not all carbs are the enemy. This is not a fad that we are proposing. Carbohydrates are here to stay and we should be glad for that. They are a priceless necessity to fuel our bodies each day. It gives a cheetah the ability to run at incredible speeds in the open savannah. What new trendy diet will there be in 10 years or even tomorrow denouncing these essential nutrients to a peon level of sorts? For us, our concern is neither here nor there. We need carbs!

Fat was the claimed villain years ago and what happened? How did fat suddenly rise to fame and power in the health and fitness world? Or did it? It should be emphasized that carbohydrates, fats, and proteins are necessary (in balanced proportions) for the human population to function at optimal efficiency. They fuel our bodies for athletics, fuel our brains, boost our energy levels, help us work better and harder, and help repair our muscles after workouts. Play it smart and choose the right group of carbs to focus on for your fuel ignition. Keep it "low" baby!

3. Are low-carb/high protein diets effective?

These diets are quite popular on the market today. You lose weight quickly on them. Isn't that what we are looking for? Losing ten pounds in two weeks?! It can't get any better than that, right? Talk to your "SUPER HEALTH" doctor and let's closely examine these diets.

Are these diets that promote rapid weight loss right for you?

Losing all of that weight so quickly? Wow! The question is, "Do you have any idea what kind of weight you are actually losing and how valuable is it for your daily, bodily functions and overall well-being?"

Because you are eliminating a high quantity of carbohydrates from your body, water is what becomes the first thing to go from your system. If you are losing more than two pounds per week, your body is drawing water (and other nutrients) from a supply found in your muscles (which contain approx. 70% water). Dehydration becomes a dangerous and likely resulting problem.

The power of water

We could spend an entire chapter denoting the importance of water for our bodies. It is the universal cleanser, flushing out our systems of daily built up toxins. It is absorbed more quickly than anything else. Everyone should consume at least 100-120 oz of water daily. When working out, you should regularly consume water throughout the session. Ideally, about half to three-quarters of a liter every 15 minutes during exercise. This allows for the sodium in your body to be carried throughout. In overall fitness, we can not emphasize that water is a star among stars and is often an overlooked muscle builder that greatly benefits you in your pursuit of a wellness lifestyle.

Another minus in eliminating those carbs from your diet

Carbohydrates are one of the three macronutrients that fuel our bodies. By eliminating a third of your caloric intake, you will surely lose the weight. What does this mean? Low carb diets tend to encourage high amounts of saturated fat being consumed to compensate for this caloric loss. This is very unhealthy and consuming these types of fats in surplus have been linked to high-blood cholesterol (LDL) levels, mineral imbalances, heart disease and many other metabolic disorders.

Glucose: the preferred source of fuel for muscle contraction

The main fuel source for exercising muscles is glycogen (chain of glucose molecules stored in the liver). This comes from carbohydrates. When you deprive your body of calories and combine this with the absence of glucose, your body will find a way to create its own glucose. Your body turns to amino acids (building blocks of protein) and begins to break down muscle tissue. If you are involved in a resistance-training program, you are in the process of trying to strengthen these muscles. This is counterproductive!

Your body will search for the needed glucose and utilize what your brain requires first and then travel to the muscle tissue. A loss of energy will result and your metabolism will slow down when the main source of fuel is being stripped from your muscle tissue. Is it worth losing a few pounds of water weight for this?

What happens when you finally get off the diet?

Sudden radical changes in your eating patterns are difficult to sustain over an extended period of time. These diets put these dieters into a quick cycle on weight loss followed by the "rebound" weight gain. Unfortunately, the water is rapidly retained as soon as the carbs are eaten and a normal diet is resumed. This is called the "yo-yo" syndrome. This sets you up for failure as you go on to the next diet.

Most diets are short-term fixes for a long-term problem. Yo-yo dieters tend to regain their weight in the abdominal region. This may be a reason why many Americans are becoming more and more obese by the day and why cancer has been on the rise and linked to obesity.

4. Is Spot Reducing Possible?

Absolutely not! On to #5. No, we are just kidding. Well, we aren't kidding that spot reducing is impossible. Here are 2 myths:

MYTH: 100 situps a day will help you lose abdominal fat.

MYTH: Inner and outer thigh machines will help you lose fat around your hip region.

As it stands to date, there isn't any scientific evidence supporting that exercise promotes fat loss in specific areas of the body. Unfortunately, we can not stay in the aerobics room for an hour doing leg lifts to attempt to shed the fat from the thighs.

What can we do then?

Genetics plays a significant role in determining where one will lose and store body fat. We must pay attention to how our parents are shaped and be conscious of where body fat is stored. This differs between genders. Most men store body fat in their abdominal region. Most women on the other hand store most of their body fat in their triceps, hips, and gluteus regions. However, we were created as functioning organisms that have the ability to MOVE. Alas, when we adhere to this sedentary lifestyle and move less, we store fat exactly where we don't want. We lose fat last where we store it first.

MEN

Fat is stored…	Fat is burned…
1. Abdominal region	1. Arms
2. Chest	2. Back
3. Back	3. Chest
4. Arms	4. Abdominal region

WOMEN

Fat is stored…	Fat is burned…
1. Hips	1. Back
2. Gluteus region	2. Abdominal region
3. Triceps	3. Triceps
4. Abdominal region	4. Gluteus region
5. Back	5. Hips

We already know the solution to this problem of having to rid our bodies of unwanted fat to gain a better appearance. Move more and eat less. As we know, the bad news is that we can not spot reduce fat, but the good news is that we can tone flabby muscles. Select one exercise for each body area and perform it for a minute. As time goes on, you will build up to 2-3 sets, three days a week. In 2-3 months, you will begin to notice a difference. With a good diet and a consistent effort in the gym, you have endless capability to achieve your goals. Go get 'em now! We have faith in you! Have faith in YOURSELF!

5. <u>Does Lifting Weights Build Big Bulky Muscles In Women?</u>

Women of all ages should be doing some form of resistance training. Building big, bulky muscles is next to impossible for women. Females, by nature, do not develop large muscles due to the fact that they do not produce enough of the male hormone, testosterone, which aids in developing that type of musculature.

Proper form when lifting weights is essential. Twelve to fifteen repetitions per set is an ideal number with a varying amount of intensity based on your individual goals. In general, shooting for 80-85% failure on the last 3 repetitions of each set will be highly effective and help you achieve that sleek physique you so desire.

Top 10 Benefits for Women That Engage in a Resistance Training Program

10. Increases bone density & prevents osteoporosis
9. Allows you to carry groceries up a flight of stairs without a loss of breath
8. Keeps you standing up straight as you age
7. Develops stronger tendons and ligaments
6. Helps to decrease body fat
5. Gives you more strength and stamina
4 Allows your clothes to fit better
3. Able to pick up your children without a risk of throwing your back out
2. Helps alter your physique
1. Increases your metabolism
The leaner your muscles are, the more calories you will burn daily.

We have seen many females alter their physiques through resistance training correctly. They comment about how much younger they look and feel. Originally, many of them believed that it was impossible to gain such a personal sense of satisfaction through this type of training. It is never too late to engage in weight training. Make it a goal to begin now and you will be able to continue doing the activities that you love for many years to come.

6. <u>Proper Form</u>

The importance of this chapter can not be overemphasized enough. The purpose of proper form is two fold: to survive and to thrive. Some exercises are more high risk than others. Avoiding any injuries in a workout is of paramount importance and can be prevented through understanding the basic fundamentals of proper form. Also, proper form is essential for smooth, muscle efficient movement especially with higher risk exercises (i.e. squats, deadlifts, military presses, etc.). Beginning your exercises with a lighter weight will be safer and easier for your body to handle. Your muscles will be able to acquire proper memory motions easier, ensuring proper form for each exercise.

What is proper form?

TOP 10 TIPS FOR PROPER FORM

10. *Get your mind in the muscle*
   -Focus on the specific muscle group that you are trying to develop.

9. *Never let the risk be greater than the reward*
   -Sacrificing form for lifting heavier weight can be a costly mistake and ultimately lead to a set of ailments possibly in tendons, ligaments, and/or joints that you can not afford. Remember, it is about the long-term benefits.

8. *Chest out & abs in*
   -Drawing your belly button inward towards your spine while extending your pectoral region outward promotes an erect spine with good posture, helping to focus on the muscle group being properly worked.

7. *Head up*
   -Your head should be up while your feet are spread slightly past shoulder width apart. Shins should also be perpendicular to the floor. This provides your body with the necessary stabilization for its ability to attack the weights properly.

6. *Stay strong on your heels*
   -This keeps everything in line from head to toe.

5. *No mercy on that muscle*
   -Maintain continuous tension on the specific muscle being worked on the way up and on the way down.

4. *Keep it slow*

-Lower the weight for twice as long as it takes to lift it. Lowering the weight (eccentric/negative motion) is the "money part" of the repetition. Muscle fibers are recruited at a greater level in this specific, force reduction portion of the lift. This is how you get stronger.

3. *The Law of Momentum does not apply*

-Keeping the tension on the muscle group worked throughout is of great importance and is your main priority. You should not be looking for an easy ride to the finish line. Keep it tight and you will gain might!

2. *Do not just "move" weight*

-This can be one of the most costly of all "no-no's". Jerking the weights around does not make you look any smarter or any stronger than your fellow gym warriors. Besides the fact that it makes you look down right silly, a muscle may be waiting in the wings for a tear. Keep it smooth and in form.

1. *Slow and steady wins the race!*

-The slower, the more concentrated on the muscle group, the more likely you will stay in proper form resulting in more efficient time use and ultimately quicker desired results.

7. <u>High Intense vs. Low Intense Cardio</u>

First, the bad news is that you must put in some time sweating it out to lose those unwanted pounds. You may ask yourself, "Do I have to spend endless hours doing cardio to burn fat?"

The answer is a resounding, NO! Participate in interval training and you will see results that you never dreamed possible. Save time and challenge yourself by mixing up the intensities of a workout in 15-20 minutes. With interval training, you can reap the benefits of an hour jog into 15-20 minutes by varying your pace and intensity.

Who can do interval training at a higher intensity?

An initial component to improving your cardiovascular health is a firm knowledge of your current level of fitness and health status. If you are a novice or just returning to the cardio arena, then you can engage in this workout starting out at a slower pace and lower heart rate and gradually progress to a more challenging level.

How does one measure their intensity?

On a scale of 1-10, honestly evaluate how hard you are working (perceived exertion). This PE number corresponds very closely with your target heart rate (ex. PE 6=target HR=60%). Your maximum heart rate (MHR) is an approximation and can be calculated by subtracting your age from 220 (ex. 40 yrs. old-MHR=180). The following chart shows where your target heart rate is for your age group.

TOP TEN TIPS HEARTRATE GUIDE

Use this as a guide when you are training aerobically on your own or at the gym. Most treadmills and bikes and elliptical crosstrainers have working heart rate monitors on the handles. We suggest buying a Polar Heart rate monitor and wearing it on your chest and you will be able to monitor your heart rate that much easier when training.

Here is how you break down your heartrate:

220 - (minus) your age x (multiply) your desired intensity

ex.- you are 40 years old

220-40=180, 180 x 75% intensity, 135 beats per minute

✧ **Low and slow 60-70%**   ✧ **Intermediate 70-80%**   ✧ **High-Intense 80-90%**

Age	Beats Per Min	Beats Per Min	Beats Per Min
18-19	121-141	141-161	161-181
20-24	119-139	139-158	158-178
25-29	116-135	135-154	154-174
30-34	113-132	132-150	150-169
35-39	110-128	128-146	146-165
40-44	107-125	125-142	142-161
45-49	104-121	121-138	138-156
50-54	101-118	118-134	134-151
55-59	98-114	114-130	130-147
60-64	95-111	111-126	126-143
65-69	92-107	107-122	122-138
70-74	89-104	104-118	118-134

You can perform interval training on many different modes. This is great because it will keep your motivation and interest levels high. Performing this training routine for 15-20 minutes can be fun. Challenge yourself utilizing a choice of fitness machines such as the standard treadmill, the stepmill, the x-trainer, the elliptical or the stationary bicycle.

What interval program is right for you?

Here are four various interval training sessions at four different fitness levels.

Beginner's Low-Impact Workout

Duration (min)	Description	Intensity (target HR)
5	treadmill	50%
8	bicycle	65%
8	elliptical climber	65%
4	treadmill	50%

Intermediate Fat-Zapper Workout

Equipment: your choice

Duration (min)	Description	Intensity (target HR)
3	warm up	50%
2	steady progress	60%
2	interval	70%
2	recovery	60%
2	interval	80%
2	recovery	60%
2	interval	80%
2	recovery	60%
2	interval	80%
2	recovery	60%
2	interval	80%
3	recovery	60%

Advanced Peak Workout

Equipment: your choice

Duration (min)	Description	Intensity (target HR)
5	warm-up	50%
3	steady progress	65%

1	higher intensity	75%
2	peak	85%
1	lower intensity	75%
2	recovery	65%
1	higher intensity	75%
2	peak	85%
1	lower intensity	75%
2	recovery	65%
1	higher intensity	75%
2	peak	85%
4	cool down	50%

Elite Fat-Burner Workout

Equipment: your choice

Duration (min)	Description	Intensity (target HR)
5	warm up	50%
2	steady progress	70%
2	high intensity	80%
1	modest recovery	70%
1	higher intensity	85%
2	modest recovery	70%
1	higher intensity	85%
2	modest recovery	70%
1	higher intensity	85%
2	modest recovery	70%
1	higher intensity	85%
2	modest recovery	70%
1	higher intensity	85%
2	modest recovery	70%
1	higher intensity	85%
2	modest recovery	70%
2	low intensity	60%
5	cool down	50%

The benefits of early morning cardio

Timing may be everything as it pertains to burning fat calories. Research has shown that cardio first thing in the morning is the best time to burn fat. It isn't due to the fact that concentrations of blood sugar and stored glycogen in muscles have plummeted overnight. Actually, those energy reserves stay fairly constant while sleeping. Your body's metabolism switches over night. Your muscles utilize fat in order to reserve glucose necessary for your brain. Ultimately, this means that fat is leaving the adipose tissue (fat cells) and travels to the muscle where it is eventually burned. Waking up early and getting in some intense cardio will cause more fat to be lost from the adipose tissue.

Top 10 benefits of early morning cardio

10) *Gets the adrenalin flowing*

-Stimulating adrenalin release increases body temperature. This will speed up your bodily functions resulting in an increase in your metabolism.

9) *Increased energy throughout the day*

-You will be burning more calories while sitting down at work due to an early morning cardio kickstart. The fat burning process is elevated for the entire day.

8) *Enjoy a "reward" meal*

-Your body is a fat-churning machine following a cardio session. When you eat breakfast following a post-cardio workout, your body takes more of the fat from the meal and delivers it to the muscles to be efficiently burned. This is rewarding to know, but also realize that you can not indulge every day. Stick to a once-a-week reward day of bacon and eggs.

7) *Shifts your biological clock*

-Habitual morning workouts will stimulate your metabolism and enhance most bodily functions throughout the day.

6) *Increases mental acuity*

-Exercise causes a release of endorphins and insulin-like growth factor I (IGF-I) that increase both mental alertness and acuity. This effect can last for at least 8 hours during the day. Following a morning workout, this will help your overall efficiency and successes at work.

5) *Builds self-discipline*

-Studies have shown that working out in the morning results in a more consistent follow through of a diet and exercise program.

4) *Helps prevent many unnecessary injuries*

-As the day wears on, the discs in our vertebrae compress and essentially we shrink (slightly). With an early morning routine, we have the least risk of injuring our back. The gravitational compression on our discs throughout the day causes a water loss, increased stiffness and less flexibility. With proper stretching following an early morning routine, we can offset many of those physical stresses on our body considering the awkward positions we can assume (in many of our jobs).

3) *Saves on your hard-earned muscle growth*

-Performing cardio on a separate day from resistance training will prevent the risk of the hormone cortisol from breaking down your muscle. To prevent muscle breakdown, before your early morning cardio, take a protein supplement high in alanine and glutamine (ex. egg proteins-high in alanine & casein (in milk)-high in glutamine).

2) *Puts you in a healthy state of mind*

-This produces multi-fold benefits at work, at the gym (workout days) and at home. Your energy levels will be much higher and your body awareness throughout the day will be enhanced.

1) *Gives you a sense of pride*

-An intense early morning cardio session sets you up with a champion's mentality feeling that you can accomplish anything. This awareness of achievement carries with you into work and throughout the day. Don't be surprised if that winning spirit rubs off on other people around you over time.

If your personal fitness objective is to take your cardiovascular levels to uncharted heights, then this is the way to go. It is the fastest and most efficient way to augment one's overall fitness level. Because time is an issue in our world and for all you working professionals, we should use it wisely and efficiently. You are working in the "moderate" to "hard" zone for a short span of time consequently obtaining maximum benefits. Good luck and hit it with a passion unparalleled!

8. The Benefits of Pilates, Yoga, & stretching

Pilates: A Whole Body Workout

Inspired by Joseph Pilates, this exercise is growing in popularity because of its many benefits. It conditions the entire body with a balanced blend of strength and flexibility training that improves posture, reduces stress and helps develop lean muscles. Several muscle groups are worked simultaneously through smooth, continuous motion with a particular concentration on strengthening the body's "inner core". This is the powerhouse of your framework including back, abdominal region and pelvic girdle region.

The focus of Pilates is quality of movement rather than quantity. Ideally, Pilates is practiced in a Pilates studio or a gym's aerobic center under the supervision of a certified Pilates instructor in a small group setting. These exercises emphasize breathing, form and posture with the goal of increasing flexibility, strength and mobility. This is a mind and body exercise performed with an internal focus, which reaps great rewards and gives you an invigorating feeling after the session.

Yoga: A Stress Buster

Yoga is a discipline that involves directing one's attention and breath focusing the mind as one assumes a series of poses. It is extremely important for improving flexibility, muscular strength, muscular endurance and stress management.

Stress is the most destructive factor in the aging process. Stress management has become a necessity in today's competitive society. Yoga is a great way to manage and combat stress through a focus and awareness of one's own breathing patterns and how to best regulate it for inner peace. Yoga postures combined with deep breathing facilitate deep relaxation and stress reduction. As with Pilates, most gyms offer Yoga classes taught by certified instructors. If your goal is to reduce stress, gain flexibility and strengthen your core, then we highly recommend engaging in either Yoga or Pilates once a week. You will be one step closer to obtaining SUPER HEALTH!

Stretching: Keep the Muscle Happy
When not to stretch:

Taking a food item right out of the freezer and trying to stretch it or starting a car that has been sitting in below freezing conditions and revving the car to perform at highway speeds are two examples of illogical actions that can result in unexpected mishaps. We, as human beings, are in many ways like a machine. We need to be warmed up before we can operate on our best functions.

It's time to warm up!

For 5-10 minutes, you can warm up on the treadmill/bike to increase blood flow to the extremities or you may choose to do a set of 20-25 standing jumping jacks to loosen up the tendons and ligaments. At this point, you can stretch out the body. Always perform static stretching, never bouncing, but rather holding a set stretch position for 10-15 seconds.

Warm up $\Rightarrow$ 5-10 minutes

Stretching ⟹ 2-3 minutes
Training ⟹ 40 minutes
Cardio ⟹ 15 minutes

Stretching between sets is also beneficial (15-30 second static stretch). It helps maintain muscular length and increase strength throughout a workout. Following your workout, stretching can help reduce onset muscle soreness caused by lactic acid buildup. Stretching transports blood to the muscles, carrying valuable nutrients (i.e. oxygen) that can be utilized.

9. <u>The Best Workout you have never done</u>

Often times, people tend to spend too much time in the gym overworking their muscles, performing too many exercises for each muscle group. Studies indicate that there is an optimal amount of time that one should concentrate his/her efforts in the gym. You need about forty minutes of resistance training no more than 4-5 days a week for optimal gain. You perform the work in the gym and your muscles increase in strength and size outside of the gym. This increase in size is called hypertrophy.

The first stage of this muscle building process is actually a muscle breakdown followed by a second stage where you must provide your muscles with sufficient rest for rebuilding, recovering and regrowing. Your time in the gym should be well spent; no more than 45 minutes. Any time spent after that is serving your muscles' a "physical injustice" to their growth and development.

Before you enter the "house of pain", you must have the mentality to attack those weights. Here is a plan of attack with a focus on the muscle. Your workouts will consist of an alternating schedule where days 1 & 3 will concentrate on upper body exercises while days 2 & 4 will focus on lower body exercises. The key to success here is (ironically) failure. No, not quitting and walking back out the door! Rather, you want to work each set performed (a group of repetitions) to muscular fatigue (99% of its potential energy) where you can not possibly push the weight another repetition with good form.

Now to the workout that you probably have never done that will ultimately result in greater efficiency in your everyday activities at work and at home. You will be pleasantly surprised to discover how well it works for you.

Day 1 Upper Body Workout (1 exercise/bodypart)

Walk for 10 minutes at a moderate pace to warm up your body
Warm up with 50 arm circles to get the shoulder muscles and joints ready for action.

Start with a light weight that you can comfortably perform 15 repetitions with (ex. Bench press-135 lbs)
Rest for 1 minute.
Choose a weight that allows you to go to failure between 8-10 repetitions (this is the "working set"). Focus and attack those weights.(ex. Bench press-225 lbs)
Right away (no rest) reduce the weight to your starting weight (Bench press-135 lbs) and perform 12 repetitions to failure.
Immediately "drop down" the weight to perform 12 repetitions to failure.(Bench press-95 lbs)
Rest for a couple of minutes and go on to the next body part repeating these steps.

*This short, intense exercise routine will keep your muscles alerted and ready to fire throughout the workout.

Provided are a list of exercises to be performed for day 1:

1. Chest (bench press)
2. Back (seated lat rows)
3. Biceps (standing barbell curls)
4. Shoulders (seated dumbbell presses)
5. Triceps (lying extensions)
6. Lower Back (extensions)

Note: Your individual strengths will dictate your starting and drop set points. As time progresses, your starting and drop set weights will increase and you will have to adjust accordingly.

There you have it. You will be out of the gym in about 42 minutes with a tremendously intense workout complete and under your belt. The following workouts will possess the same hitting power on your muscular growth and development.

Day 2-Lower Body Workout (legs)
Warmup-10 min. on the treadmill or bicycle.

* The same repetition scheme for day 1 applies here for day 2.

Provided are a list of exercises to be performed for day 2:

1. Squats
2. Lying leg curls
3. Stationary Lunges
4. Standing Calf Raises
5. Abdominal Crunches

Day 3-Upper Body Workout

Provided are a list of exercises to be performed for day 3:

1. Incline Dumbbell Press
2. Lat Pulldown
3. Side Raises
4. Standing Tricep Pressdowns

5. Seated Hammer Curls
6. Low Back Machine

Day 4- Lower Body Workout

Provided are a list of exercises to be performed for day 4:

1. Leg Press
2. Leg Extensions
3. Seated Calf Raises
4. Seated Leg Curl

This four-day workout routine will build consistent strength over a period of time. Continuity here is the key to efficiency. The goal is four days a week of workout with sufficient rest in between. After upper and lower body workouts (days 1 & 2), rest for one day before returning to the gym. Then, return for days 3 & 4 of the cycle and follow with two days of rest. Your weekly workout schedule should follow this pattern below:

Day 1	Day 2	REST DAY	Day 3	Day 4	2 REST DAYS
Upper body	Lower body		Upper body	Lower body	

You can incorporate this around your work schedule and as you can see, it is very time efficient. You are in and out of the gym in no time with outstanding benefits to follow. Three months consistently, four days a week, forty minutes a workout session, and proper rest equal significant gains in strength, energy and attitude that you never thought possible.

10. <u>Alcohol</u>

Regular drinking has substantial negative health consequences attached. Be are aware that it adversely affects our physical, emotional, and social conditions. For tip-top shape, mentality is our springboard for success or failure. So, we need a clear, coherent mind to be in full operation.

Granted that over 2/3 of Americans enjoy alcoholic beverages throughout their lifetime. But, if the goal is overall fitness achievement for your life, then some things need to be taken into serious consideration. Let's explore the facts.

The facts about alcohol

When alcohol (ethyl alcohol) is present in the body, it is carried throughout the blood stream. Enzymes in the liver metabolize the toxic chemicals of alcohol into carbon dioxide and water. Furthermore, this breakdown process is relatively slow. Alcohol acts like a diuretic stimulating your body to frequently excrete in the form of urine. Your body shifts its focus to speed up the burning of these "empty, non-nutritive" carbohydrate calories versus burning fat for energy. The result is storage of fat where you don't want it. This is where the term "beer belly syndrome" originated.

The alcohol consumed carries over to the following day and gives your body a sluggish feeling due to its working overtime. This often translates into a lack of motivation to working out, understandably so. You may be asking the question to yourself, "What if I don't get intoxicated, but occasionally drink? Will that affect my fitness and muscle-building process?"

Many studies indicate that it does not matter whether you drink occasionally or consume alcohol on a frequent basis. There is a positive correlation between these behaviors and negative effects on muscle growth. Why?

Alcohol decreases protein synthesis and increases the aging process in your cells. Your body is in a state of catabolism (break down) versus anabolism (build up), which we need for muscle growth. Excessive use or binge drinking can result in decreased levels of testosterone in men and increased levels of cortisol, which is a muscle-wasting hormone. This is also the hormone that is released when you over train.

Benefits of alcohol?

Studies have shown that for the moderate drinker, who consumes 1-2 glasses of red wine daily, the antioxidants present offer some protection against heart disease. Can you get these same benefits from something other than alcohol? Absolutely.

The disease fighting antioxidants called flavonoids in grape juice, like those in red wine, help limit the levels of LDL cholesterol that function to aid the formation of plaque on the interior of the blood vessels.

Welch's or wine?

Wine has blood-thinning properties that prevent clotting, but here is the catch. Studies have shown that this action only works when levels of alcohol are consumed high enough to declare one legally drunk. What occurs is actually damage to blood vessel tissues due to the generation of free radicals in the blood stream. This counteracts any of the benefits that red wine may offer. Research has also shown that your heart can experience the benefits from the antioxidants in grape juice for a longer period of time.

Recent studies have shown that a highly touted juice called pomegranate juice contains twice as many polyphenols (plant pigments) as red wine, helping lower the risk of various cancers, alleviate various menopausal symptoms, reduce blood pressure, and clear the bloodstream from unwanted cholesterol in addition to other numerous benefits.

As is clearly evident, there are alternatives to consuming alcohol in helping your overall fitness and health status. The next time that you are out, think about the negative consequences of alcohol and weigh your options carefully.

CHAPTER 9

SUPPLEMENTS FROM A-Z

Supplement/Our Rating	Benefits Claimed	Top Tip
1.Antioxidants **(9.5)**	1. helps minimize amount of free radicals in the body 2. helps prevent fatigue and muscle damage during exercise 3. strengthens immune system	combined w/ a multi-vitamin, you will destroy free radicals
2. *Branch chain amino acids (BCAAs), valine, leucine, isoleucine* **(7.5)**	1. fuel for muscles while training 2. prevents catabolism during intense training	if your workouts are intense, you will benefit from extra BCAA's
3. *Caffeine* **(8.0)**	1. most widely consumed natural drug in the world 2. enhances mental alertness 3. increases endurance in events lasting longer than 20 minutes	in moderation; acts as a diuretic; benefits best pre-workout
4. *Conjugated linoleic acid (CLA)* **(6.5)**	1. aids in weight loss 2. may lower risk of heart disease 3. may positively help body composition	CLA is found in beef (choose lean sources and dairy fats-ex. 1 egg yolk a day)
5. *Chromium Picolinate* **(3.5)**	1. helps aid glucose metabolism	side effects include upset stomach & kidney damage

6. *Coenzyme Q-10* **(3.0)**	1. enhances ATP production	lacking significant evidence & studies showing benefits
7. *Creatine* **(9.0)**	1. improves strength, power, recovery 2. increases muscle size 3. increases water retention in muscle	try taking for 3 weeks on, 1 week off; studies to date have not shown any negative side effects when taken responsibly
8. *Echinacea* **(6.0)**	1. reduces duration of colds 2. boosts immune system	no regulated manufacturing standards; if you have a cold, bump up your vit. C an extra 1000 mg. every 2 hrs.
9. *Essential Fatty Acids* *(omega 3-, omega 6, flaxseed) (EFAs)* **(10.0)**	1. assures proper heart function 2. helps maximize testosterone production	found in fish; have fish 2 to 3 times a week-1000 mg EFAs
10. *Ginkgo biloba* **(4.5)**	1. improves blood flow, memory, & mental focus (potentially)	contains antioxidant properties that are beneficial to blood flow and neural function; not enough significant research to validate its effect
11. *Ginseng* **(5.0)**	1. helps body adapt to higher stress levels 2. increases endurance 3. improves mental focus & energy	combined w/ ginkgo may improve memory & mental focus
12. *Glucosamine/ Chondroitin* **(7.5)**	1. possible treatment for arthritis 2. possible rehab for cartilage 3. strengthens joints	take immediately after training & before bed for 1 month to see if this product works for you

13. *Glutamine* **(10.0)**	1. helps enhance immune system 2. causes extra growth hormone release 3. enhances cell volume in muscles 4. helps in high-stress situations	take 5-10 grams daily
14. *HMB* **(5.0)**	1. increases body's ability to build muscle and burn fat in response to intense exercise	not enough bang for $
15. *Melatonin* **(8.5)**	1. all-natural sleep aid w/ out side effects of prescription sleep aids 2. strengthens immune system 3. reduces free radicals in body	best if taken 30 min. before bed (pregnant, nursing women should not take this)
16. *Meal replacement powders (MRPs)* **(9.5)**	1. quick, healthy source of quality protein w/ out excess calories 2. the ultimate post-workout fuel source 3. economical and packed w/ nutrients	avoid the ones high in sugar/corn syrup; look for ones w/ maltodextrin
17. *Nitric oxide* **(7.5)**	1. continuous muscle pump that lasts several hours post-workout 2. increases muscle growth 3. increases recovery & stamina 4. increases vascularity	this will provide a great pump while working out, but the actual muscle benefits are not known at this time
18. *Protein powders* **(9.0)**	1. high bio-availability level of protein, important for recovery & building muscle 2. good post-workout fuel source 3. low-caloric protein source	MRPs have more nutrients than protein powders; these are a good second choice; protein is not a supplement; try to consume all of your protein from food sources; choose from whey products
19. *Pyruvate* **(3.5)**	1. helps breakdown carbs for energy 2. helps obese people lose weight	very expensive; if one consumes adequate carbs, exercises regularly, then pyruvate is naturally manufactured in the body w/ out any need for supplementation

20. *Saw Palmetto* (**4.0**)	1. Men over 50: it helps prevent prostate enlargement	potential risk is not known; no regulated manufacturing standards for these compounds
21. *Synephrine* (**7.5**)	1. increases metabolism 2. fat burner (promotes weight loss) 3. increases energy levels 4. ephedra's safer little brother w/ out the side effects	safer than ephedra; use in moderation and consult w/ doctor
22. *Tyrosine* (**8.0**)	1. all-natural stimulant 2. improves mental focus & concentration	take 2 grams 30 min. before training to feel the difference
23. *Zinc, magnesium aspartate (ZMA)* (**7.0**)	1. increases testosterone & HGH levels in men 2. enhances recovery while you sleep	best if taken 30 min. before bedtime; will provide a great night's sleep

CHAPTER 10

TIP TOP TERMS

1. 5/5 RULE

WHEN PURCHASING BREAKFAST CEREALS, LOOK ON THE NUTRITION LABEL AND MAKE SURE THAT THERE ARE 5 GRAMS OR LESS OF SUGAR AND 5 GRAMS OR MORE OF FIBER.

2. ACTIVITY LEVEL

THIS IS A LEVEL OF 1-10 (1-LEAST ACTIVE & 10-MOST ACTIVE). WE DISCUSS HOW YOU CAN MAKE THIS LOW OR HIGH ACTIVITY LEVEL AT YOUR JOB WORK FOR YOU.

3. ALL-STAR FOODS

THE FOODS YOU WANT TO EAT AT LEAST 80% OF YOUR WAKING EXISTENCE TO ACHIEVE A SUPER HEALTH STATE.

4. CHALLENGES

THE HUMAN BODY IS MADE TO RESPOND TO THE CALL OF DUTY. DO SOMETHING EACH DAY THAT TAKES YOU UP A LEVEL AND PUSHES YOU TO BETTER YOUR MIND, BODY, AND SOUL. SET YOUR STANDARDS HIGH AND CONTINUE TO ACCEPT THESE CHALLENGES AS THEY COME.

5. CIRCUIT TRAINING

A GREAT WAY TO DO YOUR WEIGHT RESISTANCE TRAINING. PERFORM A CERTAIN AMOUNT OF AN EXERCISE INCORPORATING THE WHOLE BODY WITH LITTLE TO NO REST IN BETWEEN EXERCISES KEEPING YOUR HEART RATE ELEVATED THROUGHOUT. THIS IS A GOOD, CHALLENGING WORKOUT THAT WILL BURN A GREAT AMOUNT OF CALORIES WHILE AND AFTER WORKING OUT.

6. COMPETITION

REMEMBER THAT SOMEONE IS ALWAYS OUT THERE WORKING HARDER THAN YOU. ALWAYS SET YOUR GOALS HIGH AND NEVER SETTLE FOR SECOND. ENGAGE IN QUALITY, HEALTHY COMPETITIVE EVENTS THAT YOU CAN FIT INTO YOUR SCHEDULE AND LIFESTYLE.

7. CONSISTENCY

NONE OF THE OTHER TOOLS MATTER IF YOU ARE NOT CONSISTENT IN YOUR DIET & EXERCISE PROGRAM. THIS IS A KEY INGREDIENT TO OBTAINING LONG-TERM GOALS.

8. DISCIPLINE

EVERY GREAT LEADER HAS THE ABILITY TO TAKE CONTROL OF HIS/HER ACTIONS IN MOST (IF NOT ALL) ASPECTS OF LIFE. WITH EACH DISPLAY OF SELF-DISCIPLINE, YOU WILL REALIZE THAT YOU HAVE THE ULTIMATE POWER TO ACHIEVE YOUR GOALS.

9.ENERGY LEVELS

THE AMOUNT OF MENTAL & PHYSICAL STRENGTH THROUGHOUT THE DAY CAN FLUCTUATE. TIPS ARE PROVIDED FOR A MORE STABLE, WELL-BALANCED ENERGY LEVEL.

10. FAILURE %

FOR EVERY REPETITION PERFORMED DURING THE WORKING SETS, YOUR GOAL IS TO REACH A CERTAIN LEVEL OF MUSCLE FATIGUE. 100% FAILURE IS THE POINT AT WHICH YOU CAN NOT LIFT THE WEIGHT ANOTHER REPETITION. GOING TO 100 % FAILURE ALL OF THE TIME IS VERY HARD TO DO WITHOUT A SPOTTER AND WITHOUT RISKING GETTING INJURED. IT SHOULD ONLY BE DONE IF YOU ARE AN ADVANCED TRAINEE. YOU HAVE TO KNOW YOUR BODY AND BE ABLE TO TAKE IT TO FAILURE WITH GOOD FORM OF COURSE. % FAILURE CHANGES AS YOU GET STRONGER. YOU MAY BE ONLY ABLE TO PERFORM 7 REPS OF AN EXERCISE AT A CERTAIN WEIGHT AND THEN FAIL ON THE 8TH REP (100% FAILURE). (NOTE: THE 4TH REP OF THAT SET WOULD EQUAL ABOUT 50% FAILURE)

11. HIGH RISK EXERCISES

SQUATS, DEADLIFTS, DIPS, BENCH PRESS CAN ALL BE CLASSIFIED AS HIGH RISK EXERICES AND YOU SHOULD ALWAYS BE CAREFUL OF YOUR FORM AND NEVER SACRIFICE THIS OR ELSE YOU COULD GET SERIOUSLY INJURED AND PUT A MAJOR BUMP IN

THE ROAD FOR YOU. EVERY EXERCISE COULD BE HIGH RISK IF YOU DO NOT MONITOR YOUR FORM.

12. INTENSITY

BRINGING THE FIRE, FLARE, AND PASSION INTO YOUR WORKOUTS CAN MAKE A HUGE DIFFERENCE ON YOUR OVERALL PERFORMANCE. THESE DAILY ACCOMPLISH-MENTS ADD UP TO GREATER SUCCESSES DOWN THE ROAD.

13. INTERVALS

THIS IS A GREAT, ADVANCED METHOD OF TRAINING. THIS IS WHERE YOU PERFORM A CARDIOVASCULAR EXERCISE AND PROCEED AT A CERTAIN LEVEL/ SPEED FOR A DES-IGNATED TIME. DURING THE EXERCISE, THE INTENSITY IS INCREASED BRINGING YOUR HEART RATE UP HIGHER. THIS IS THE MOST EFFICIENT WAY TO TAKE YOUR AEROBIC CONDITIONING TO ANOTHER LEVEL.

14. MENTAL EXERCISE

MANY PROFESSIONS REQUIRE A GREAT DEAL OF MENTAL STAMINA THROUGHOUT THE DAY. WE SHOW YOU HOW YOU CAN JUMPSTART YOUR PERFORMANCES AT WORK DURING THE DAY MAINTAINING FOCUS AND CONCENTRATION.

15. MIND IN THE MUSCLE

WHEN WORKING ON A SPECIFIC BODY PART DURING YOUR WORKOUT, FOCUS YOUR MIND SOLELY ON THE MUSCLE YOU ARE TRAINING. PUT 100 % FOCUS INTO THAT AREA IN ORDER TO GET THE MOST BENEFIT.

16. MODERATION

MAINTAINING A CONSISTENT DESIRED LEVEL IN YOUR DIET & EXERCISE.

17. MOTIVATION

IF THERE IS A WILL, THERE IS A WAY! LISTEN TO TAPES, BE AROUND PEOPLE WHO HAVE SIMILAR AMBITIONS AND GOALS LIKE YOU. THE MIND ACTS ON WHAT IT BELIEVES.

18. MOVING AND GROOVING

THESE ARE WAYS THAT YOU CAN MOVE MORE THROUGHOUT THE DAY BASED ON YOUR PROFESSION. MOVING MORE IS A KEY COMPONENT FOR BURNING THOSE EXCESS CALORIES THROUGHOUT THE DAY AND STAYING FIT.

19. OBSTACLES

WE ENCOUNTER DAILY HURDLES EVERYDAY. WE SHOW YOU HOW TO DESTROY THESE OBSTACLES AND NOT TO LET THEM DETER YOU FROM HITTING YOUR GOALS. YOU WILL ENCOUNTER THESE BUMPS IN THE ROAD. THESE ARE ALL PART OF THE WONDERFUL STORYBOOK THAT MAKES YOUR JOURNEY TO SUCCESS THAT MUCH MORE INTERESTING.

20. OVERALL WELLNESS

HAVING AN OPTIMUM LEVEL OF BOTH MENTAL STRENGTH & PHYSICAL STRENGTH.

21. PEAK POTENTIAL

YOUR HIGHEST LEVEL (OR CLOSE TO IT) OF POTENTIAL ACCOMPLISHMENT MENTALLY & PHYSICALLY.

22. PLYOMETRIC POWER.

A WORKOUT FOR THE ADVANCED ATHLETE. THE WORKOUT RECRUITS MANY FAST TWITCH MUSCLE FIBERS AND HELPS YOU TAKE YOUR TRAINING TO ANOTHER LEVEL. THESE ARE EXERCISES WHERE THE MUSCLE IS CONTRACTED ECCENTRICALLY, AND THEN IMMEDIATELY CONCENTRICALLY. THIS IS WHERE THE MUSCLE IS STRETCHED BEFORE IT IS CONTRACTED. EX.- PUSHUPS WITH A CLAP IN BETWEEN EACH PUSHUP.

23.RESISTANCE TRAINING

A WEIGHT TRAINING PROGRAM THAT INCORPORATES WORKOUTS TO BUILD MUSCLE STRENGTH/ENDURANCE.

24. REWARD DAY

IF YOU ARE ON POINT 90%-100% OF THE TIME DURING THE WEEK WITH YOUR DIET, FEEL FREE TO EAT YOUR MOST DESIRED FOODS FOR A DAY OUT OF THE WEEK.

25. SITTING

SOME PROFESSIONS REQUIRE A GREAT DEAL OF THIS, WHICH MAKES YOU MOVE LESS AND YOU KNOW THAT YOU HAVE TO MOVE MORE IN ORDER TO ACHIEVE SUPER HEALTH. WE SHOW YOU HOW YOU CAN MOVE MORE EVEN WHILE YOU ARE SITTING IN THESE PROFESSIONS.

26.SKIPPING MEALS

A BIG 'NO,NO' WHEN IT COMES TO YOUR NUTRITION. SMALL MEALS EATEN FREQUENTLY THROUGHOUT THE DAY HAVE PROVEN TO STIMULATE YOUR METABOLISM AND BURN CALORIES AT AN ELEVATED RATE THROUGHOUT THE DAY. GOING TOO LONG WITHOUT EATING A SMALL MEAL WILL SET YOU UP FOR LOW ENERGY LEVELS IN THE GYM AND AT YOUR WORKPLACE.

27. STRESS LEVEL

THIS IS A LEVEL OF 1-10 RATING (1-LEAST STRESSED 10- MOST STRESSED) THAT GAUGES THE STRESS LEVEL THAT EACH PROFESSION HAS AND HOW YOU CAN EFFECTIVELY REDUCE IT. THIS PLAYS A SIGNIFICANT ROLE IN YOUR CUSTOMIZED PROGRAM.

28. SUPER HEALTH

EXERCISING, EATING AND SLEEPING YOUR WAY TO THE BEST "YOU" IS THE GOAL OF THIS BOOK. OUR BOOK IS DESIGNED FOR YOU, SO THAT IF YOU FOLLOW THE TIPS AND YOUR CUSTOMIZED PROGRAMS WE DESIGN FOR YOU IN YOUR PROFESSION, THEN YOU WILL ACHIEVE THIS STATE OF SUPER HEALTH.

29. SUPERMANS

A GREAT LOW BACK EXERCISE. LYING FULL PRONE ON YOUR STOMACH. KEEP YOUR ARMS IN FRONT OF YOU STRAIGHT OUT AND RAISE YOUR ARMS AND LEGS UP AT THE SAME TIME AND HOLD FOR 3-5 SECONDS REPEATING A GIVEN NUMBER OF REPETITIONS.

30. SUPERSETS

2 EXERCISES DONE BACK TO BACK WITH NO REST IN BETWEEN EXERCISES. THE EXERCISES ARE USUALLY FOR THE SAME BODYPART.

WORD FROM THE AUTHORS

Do it right! For overall, long-term fitness, wellness, and SUPER HEALTH there aren't any quick fixes. If it were easy, then everyone would do it. We are not asking you to run miles a day and watch exactly what you eat. We realize that you are human and that you have lives just like everyone else. Throughout this book, we have discussed a set of various tips for improving your health and exercise in a time frame that is manageable. We have documented 20 different professions and provided cross-referencing for you to customize a plan that works best for your personal needs. Stay focused, disciplined to the best of your ability, and follow these recommended tips for tip-top shape. Your body will begin to adapt to your workouts and you will need to adjust accordingly by using our tips to continue your upward progression towards SUPER HEALTH. We provide you with the knowledge and understanding to achieve your wellness goals. Now, the sky is the limit for you. Take what we have provided and fly with it! We have personally witnessed it work for others at all levels including ourselves and the goals that we have personally ascertained have been incredible, often times beyond our wildest dreams. Along the ride, stay strong mentally, physically, and emotionally. There will always be bumps and curves in the road. That is why it is called life. Take your obstacles and turn them into opportunities. Your perception on life controls your results. Believe that our tips will greatly help you. Implement them into your life and remain patient and focused and results will follow. This will work for anyone at any level. We are proud of each and every one of you! Good luck!

ABOUT THE AUTHORS

Matthew DeLeo has been a professional fitness instructor for nearly 10 years and has worked with clients as old as 87 and as young as 16. He has worked with special needs children in helping them discover their own capabilities through exercise and fitness. Mr. DeLeo specializes in exercise & physiology and has trained over 300 people including athletes, stars, and successful business people, alike. He has over 10 nationally accredited certifications in the Health and Fitness field including National Academy of Sports Medicine, Resistance Training Specialist and Apex Nutrition. He has also been featured as a top fitness model in many publications, catalogs, and billboards over the years such as Men's Exercise, Natural Bodybuilding, Spongex Aquatic Fitness Equipment, and Eastern Mountain Sports to name a few. Furthermore, Mr. DeLeo is a professional championship natural bodybuilder at both state and national levels. He won the title as Mr. Connecticut 2001 and Mr. USA Natural Middleweight 2004 in Tarrytown, NY.

Douglas Haddad graduated magna cum laude from Central Connecticut State University with a bachelor's degree in biology/secondary education and a master's degree in biology. He has taught "Chemistry of Nutrition" at Central Connecticut State University and worked alongside many professors in nutrition, exercise, and physiology research. Haddad is certified by the National Academy of Sports Medicine as a Performance Enhancement Specialist for elite athletes. He was a member of a statewide cardio-kickboxing championship team. Haddad enjoys practicing Tai Chi Ch'uan on a regular basis.

<u>TESTIMONIALS</u>

My transition from Connecticut to New York City to break into the acting scene called for a change of pace and didn't allow much time for me to work out as much as I did in the past. Doug Haddad designed a simple exercise and nutrition plan that helped me stay in great shape despite my hectic schedule. My energy level feels high throughout the day and my confidence is soaring. I feel great! I strongly feel that the customized plans in this book will work for anyone's schedule.

-Chris Holmes, actor

Doug Haddad has customized a lifestyle plan in which I have lost 12 pounds in the past 3 months, without any exercise due to a back injury, by changing my eating habits and never feeling hungry. I can confidently say that my motivation and confidence are very high. I have tried so many diets before that have worked temporarily. This is a lifestyle plan that will work for anyone!

-Debora Taylor, school guidance counselor

We have incorporated the principles in this book and have seen tremendous physical and mental improvements. We thank Doug for his advice about how to live a healthier lifestyle.

-John Pleva & Rob Santiago, custodians

I can't begin to describe the positive effects that this book has had on my life.

-Thomas McNamee, M.D.

I have shed 15 lbs and increased my energy and strength to all new heights. I feel 10 years younger and 10 times stronger. This book is a must read for working professionals who want revitalization.

-Daniel Picagli, police officer